The Mediterranean Way

Health and Tasty Recipes to Discover New Foods and
Boost Your Taste

I0146023

America Best Recipes

Table of contents

Salsa Rice

Preparation Time: 10 minutes

Cooking Time: 15 minutes

Servings: 6

Ingredients:

- 9 oz long grain rice
- 4 cups chicken stock
- 1 cup of salsa
- 2 tbsp. avocado oil

Directions:

1. Mix chicken stock and rice in the saucepan.
2. Cook the rice for 15 minutes on medium heat.
3. Then cool it to the room temperature and mix with avocado oil and salsa.

Nutrition:

Calories: 109;

Protein: 12.3g;

Carbs: 7.4g;

Fat: 6.3g

Seafood Rice

Preparation Time: 10 minutes

Cooking Time: 30 minutes

Servings: 4

Ingredients:

- ½ cup seafood mix, frozen
- ½ cup of long grain rice
- 3 cups of water
- 1 tbsp. olive oil
- ½ tsp. ground coriander

Directions:

1. Boil the rice with water for 15-18 minutes or until it soaks all water.
2. Then heat olive oil in the saucepan.
3. Add seafood mix and ground coriander. Cook the ingredients for 10 minutes on low heat.
4. Then add rice, stir well, and cook for 5 minutes more.

Nutrition:

Calories: 73;

Protein: 12.3g;

Carbs: 3.4g;

Fat: 6.3g

Vegetarian Pilaf

Preparation Time: 10 minutes

Cooking Time: 30 minutes

Servings: 6

Ingredients:

- 1 cup of long grain rice
- 2 cups of water
- 1 carrot, grated
- 2 tbsp. olive oil
- 1 tbsp. dried dill
- ½ tsp. dried mint
- ½ tsp. salt

Directions:

1. Boil rice with water for 15 minutes on medium heat.
2. Meanwhile, melt the olive oil and add the carrot.
3. Roast the carrot for 10 minutes or until it is soft.
4. Then add dried dill, mint, and cooked rice.
5. Carefully stir the pilaf and cook for 5 minutes.

Nutrition:

Calories: 123;

Protein: 10.3g;

Carbs: 2.4g;

Fat: 6.3g

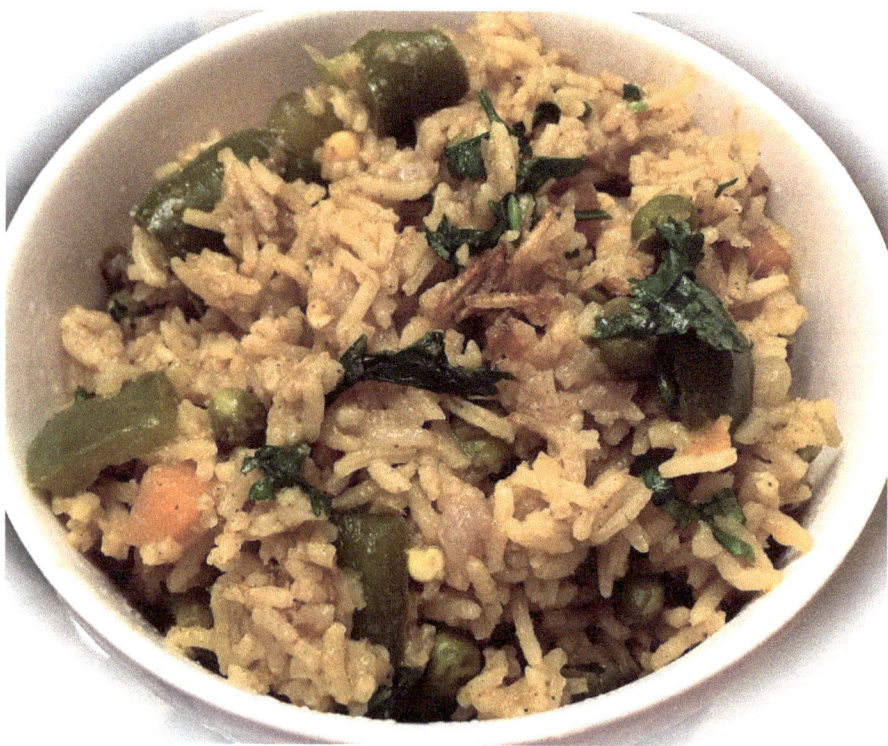

Rice Rolls

Preparation Time: 15 minutes

Cooking Time: 35 minutes

Servings: 6

Ingredients:

- 4 white cabbage leaves
- 4 oz ground chicken
- ½ tsp. garlic powder
- ¼ cup of long grain rice, cooked
- ½ cup chicken stock
- ½ cup tomatoes, chopped

Directions:

1. In the bowl, mix ground chicken, garlic powder, and rice.
2. Then put the rice mixture on every cabbage leaf and roll.
3. Arrange the rice rolls in the saucepan.
4. Add chicken stock and tomatoes and close the lid.
5. Cook the rice rolls for 35 minutes on low heat.

Nutrition:

Calories: 69;

Protein: 12.3g;

Carbs: 3.4g;

Fat: 6.3g

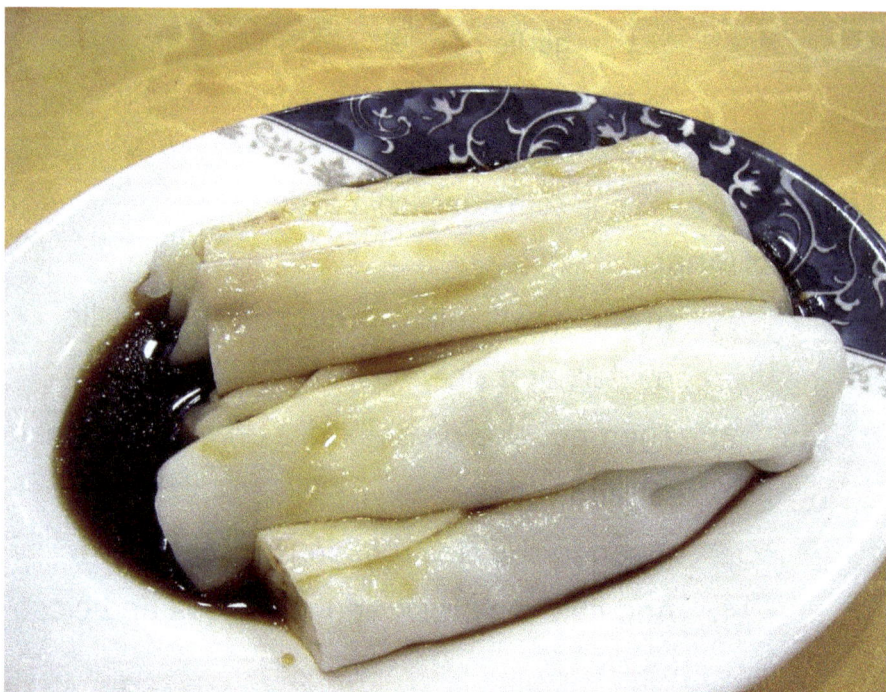

Rice Stew with Squid

Preparation Time: 10 minutes

Cooking Time: 30 minutes

Servings: 6

Ingredients:

- 5 oz long grain rice
- 4 oz squid, sliced
- 1 jalapeno pepper, chopped
- ½ cup tomatoes, chopped
- 1 onion, diced
- 2 cups chicken stock
- 1 tbsp. avocado oil

Directions:

1. Roast the onion with avocado oil in the skillet for 3-4 minutes or until the onion is light brown.
2. Add squid, jalapeno pepper, and tomatoes.
3. Cook the ingredients for 7 minutes.
4. Then cook rice with water for 15 minutes.
5. Add cooked rice in the squid mixture, stir, and cook for 3 minutes more.

Nutrition:

Calories: 153;

Protein: 12.3g;

Carbs: 3.4g;

Fat: 6.3g

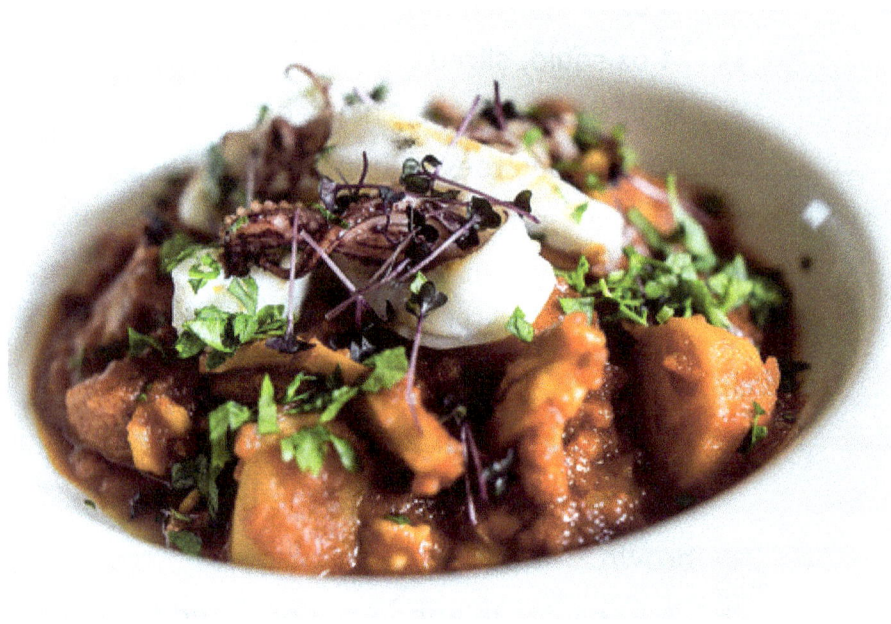

Creamy Millet

Preparation Time: 10 minutes

Cooking Time: 10 minutes

Servings: 6

Ingredients:

- ½ cup millet
- 1 oz cream cheese
- ¼ tsp. salt
- 1.5 cup hot water

Directions:

1. Mix hot water and millet in the saucepan.
2. Boil it for 8 minutes on low heat.
3. Add cream cheese and salt.
4. Carefully stir the cooked millet.

Nutrition:

Calories: 53;

Protein: 12.3g;

Carbs: 3.4g;

Fat: 6.3g

Oatmeal Cakes

Preparation Time: 15 minutes

Cooking Time: 7 minutes

Servings: 4

Ingredients:

- ½ cup oatmeal
- 1 egg, beaten
- 1 carrot, grated
- 1 tbsp. olive oil
- 1 tsp. flax meal

Directions:

1. Put oatmeal, egg, grated carrot, and flax meal in the blender. Blend the mixture well.
2. Then heat olive oil in the skillet.
3. Make the medium size cakes from the oatmeal mixture and cook for 3 minutes per side on medium heat.

Nutrition:

Calories: 63;

Protein: 12.3g;

Carbs: 3.4g;

Fat: 6.3g

Yogurt Buckwheat

Preparation Time: 5 minutes

Cooking Time: 13 minutes

Servings: 2

Ingredients:

- ½ cup buckwheat
- 1.5 cup chicken stock
- 1 tbsp. plain yogurt

Directions:

1. Put all ingredients in the saucepan and close the lid.
2. Cook the meal for 13 minutes on low heat or until the buckwheat soaks all liquid.
3. Carefully stir the cooked meal.

Nutrition:

Calories: 69;

Protein: 12.3g;

Carbs: 3.4g;

Fat: 6.3g

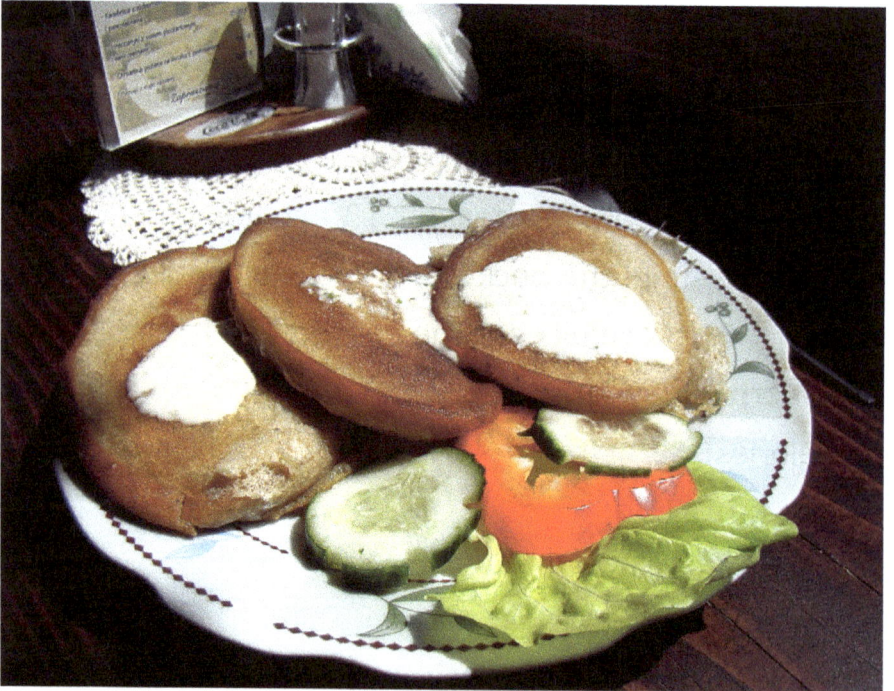

Halloumi Buckwheat Bowl

Preparation Time: 10 minutes

Cooking Time: 15 minutes

Servings: 4

Ingredients:

- 1 cup buckwheat
- cups chicken stock
- 4 oz halloumi cheese
- 1 tbsp. olive oil
- ½ tsp. dried thyme

Directions:

1. Mix chicken stock and buckwheat in the saucepan, bring to boil and cook for 7 minutes on medium heat.
2. After this, sprinkle the halloumi cheese with olive oil and dried thyme.
3. Grill it for 2 minutes per side or until the cheese is light brown.
4. Then put the cooked buckwheat in the bowls.
5. Chop the cheese roughly and top the buckwheat with it.

Nutrition:

Calories: 93;

Protein: 12.3g;

Carbs: 3.4g;

Fat: 6.3g

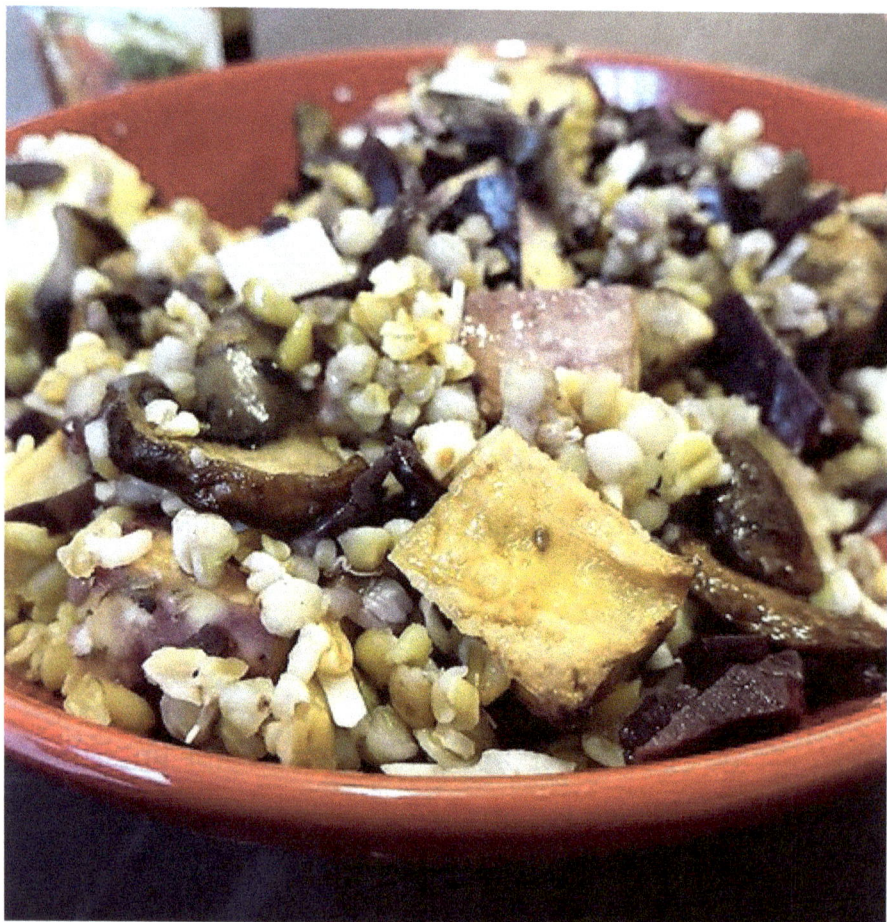

Aromatic Green Millet

Preparation Time: 10 minutes

Cooking Time: 7 minutes

Servings: 5

Ingredients:

- 1 cup millet
- 2 cups of water
- 4 tbsp. pesto sauce
- ¼ tsp. cayenne pepper

Directions:

1. Mix water and millet in the saucepan and boil for 7 minutes.
2. Then add cayenne pepper and pesto sauce.
3. Stir the millet until homogenous and green.

Nutrition:

Calories: 205;

Protein: 5.3g;

Carbs: 4.4g;

Fat: 7.3g

Quinoa with Pumpkin

Preparation Time: 5 minutes

Cooking Time: 20 minutes

Servings: 6

Ingredients:

- ½ cup pumpkin, cubed
- 1 tbsp. lemon juice
- 1 tsp. liquid honey
- 1 cup quinoa
- 2 cups of water
- ¼ cup of organic almond milk

Directions:

1. Put almond milk and pumpkin in the saucepan.
2. Add lemon juice and water.
3. Cook the pumpkin for 10 minutes.
4. Then add quinoa and cook the meal for 10 minutes.
5. Remove the cooked meal from the heat, add liquid honey, and stir well.

Nutrition:

Calories: 177;

Protein: 6.3g;

Carbs: 4.7g;

Fat: 5.3g

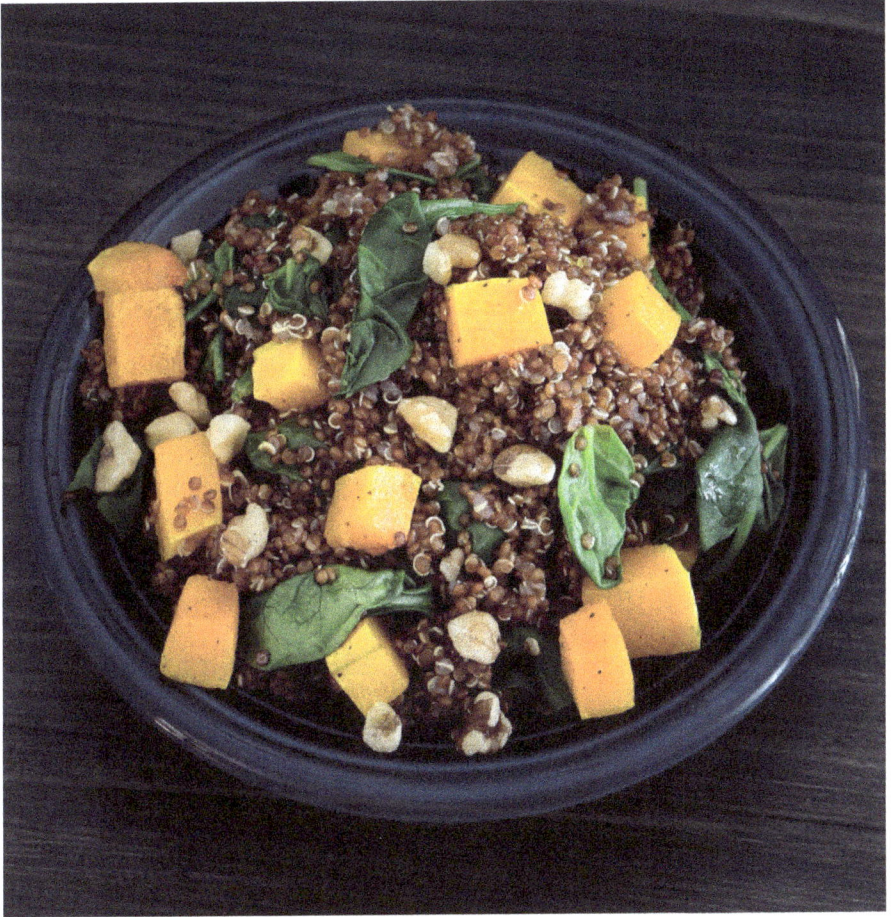

Almond Quinoa

Preparation Time: 5 minutes

Cooking Time: 4 minutes

Servings: 4

Ingredients:

- 1 cup quinoa
- 2 cups of water
- 1 cup organic almond milk
- ½ cup strawberries, sliced
- 1 tbsp. honey

Directions:

1. Pour water and milk in the saucepan and bring to boil.
2. Add quinoa and cook it for 12 minutes.
3. Then cool the cooked quinoa and add honey. Stir.
4. Transfer the quinoa in the bowls and top with strawberries.

Nutrition:

Calories: 193;

Protein: 6.3g;

Carbs: 3.4g;

Fat: 3.3g

Spring Rolls with Quinoa

Preparation Time: 10 minutes

Cooking Time: 1 minutes

Servings: 8

Ingredients:

- 8 rice pepper wraps
- 1 cup quinoa, cooked
- 1 carrot, cut into strips
- 1 cup lettuce leaves
- 1 tbsp. olive oil

Directions:

1. Make the rice pepper wraps wet.
2. Then put the cooked quinoa on every rice pepper wrap.
3. Add carrot and lettuce leaves and wrap them into the rolls.
4. Brush every roll with olive oil and put it in the hot skillet.
5. Roast the spring rolls for 20 seconds per side.

Nutrition:

Calories: 257;

Protein: 6.3g;

Carbs: 3.4g;

Fat: 6.3g

Mushroom Quinoa Skillet

Preparation Time: 10 minutes

Cooking Time: 25 minutes

Servings: 6

Ingredients:

- 1 cup mushrooms, sliced
- ½ cup of water
- 1 tbsp. olive oil
- 1 tsp. Italian seasonings
- ½ cup quinoa
- ½ cup organic almond milk
- ¼ tsp. dried thyme

Directions:

1. Roast mushrooms with olive oil in the saucepan for 10 minutes.
2. Then stir them well, add Italian seasonings, dried thyme, and quinoa.
3. Add almond milk and water.
4. Close the lid and simmer the meal for 15 minutes. Stir it from time to time to avoid burning.

Nutrition:

Calories: 12;

Protein: 3.3g;

Carbs: 3.4g;

Fat: 6.3g

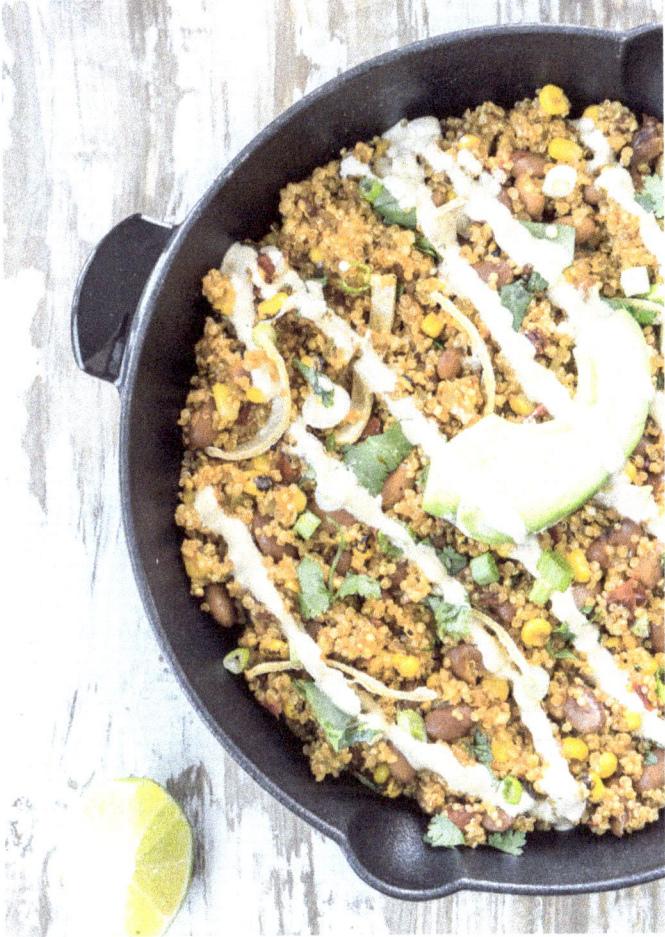

Strawberry Quinoa Bowl

Preparation Time: 15 minutes

Cooking Time: 0 minutes

Servings: 8

Ingredients:

- 2 ½ cup quinoa, cooked
- ¼ cup strawberries, roughly chopped
- ½ cup fresh spinach, chopped
- 2 pecans, chopped
- 1 tbsp. balsamic vinegar
- 1 tsp. avocado oil

Directions:

1. Mix quinoa, fresh spinach, and pecans in the big bowl.
2. Then add strawberries and avocado oil.
3. Gently shake the mixture and transfer in the serving bowls.
4. Sprinkle every serving with a small amount of balsamic vinegar.

Nutrition:

Calories: 283;

Protein: 8.3g;

Carbs: 3.4g;

Fat: 6.3g

Quinoa Meatballs

Preparation Time: 15 minutes

Cooking Time: 30 minutes

Servings: 6

Ingredients:

- ½ cup quinoa, cooked
- ½ cup ground pork
- 1 tbsp. chives, chopped
- 1 egg, beaten
- 1 tbsp. sesame seeds
- 1 tsp. chili flakes
- 1 cup tomato juice

Directions:

1. In the bowl mi quinoa, ground pork, chives, egg, sesame seeds, and chili flakes.
2. Then make the small meatballs and put them in the baking pan.
3. Top the meatballs with tomato juice and cook in the preheated to 375F oven for 30 minutes.

Nutrition:

Calories: 177;

Protein: 16.3g;

Carbs: 3.4g;

Fat: 6.3g

Stir-Fried Farro

Preparation Time: 10 minutes

Cooking Time: 8minutes

Servings: 4

Ingredients:

- 1 cup farro, cooked
- 1 egg, beaten
- 1 tbsp. olive oil
- ½ tsp. chili flakes

Directions:

1. Heat olive oil and egg beaten egg.
2. Cook it for 1 minute and then stir it carefully.
3. Add cooked farro and chili flakes.
4. Fry the meal for 7 minutes. Stir it from time to time.

Nutrition:

Calories: 196;

Protein: 6.3g;

Carbs: 3.4g;

Fat: 6.3g

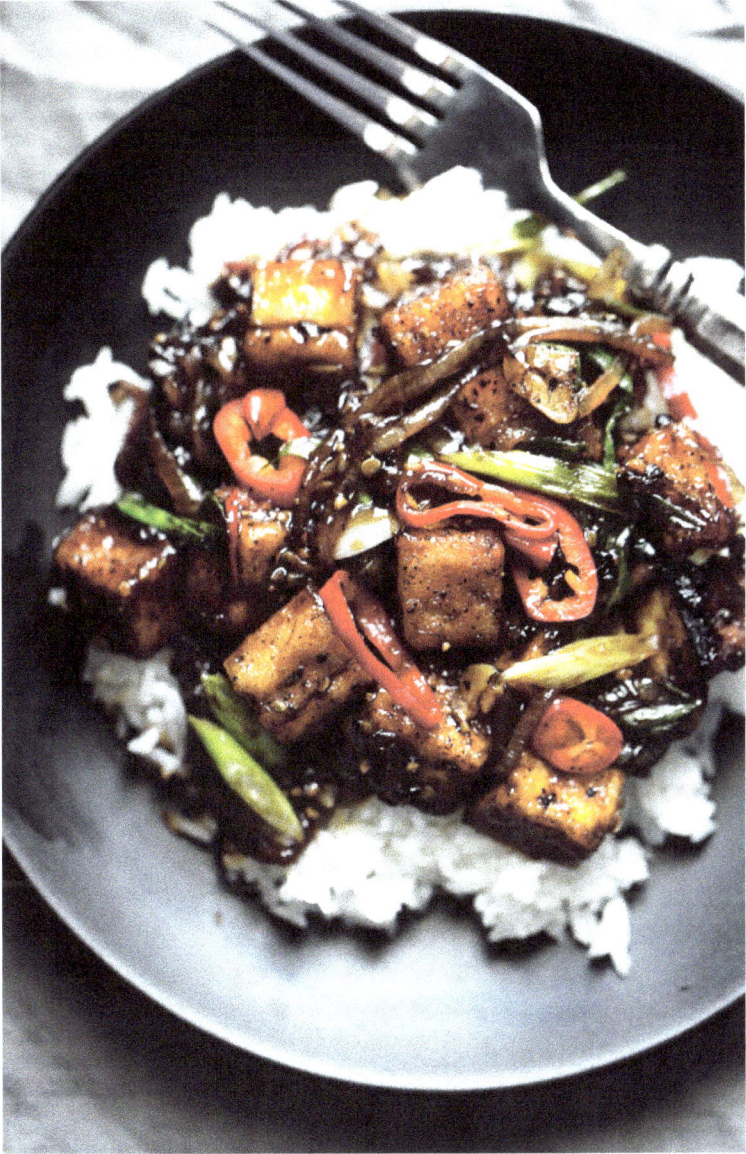

Quick Farro Skillet

Preparation Time: 10 minutes

Cooking Time: 15 minutes

Servings: 6

Ingredients:

- 2 oz fresh spinach, chopped
- 2 oz asparagus, chopped
- 1/3 cup farro, cooked
- 1 tbsp. olive oil
- ½ tsp. curry powder

Directions:

1. Line the skillet with baking paper.
2. Put all ingredients in the prepared skillet, flatten them gently and transfer in the preheated to 365°F oven.
3. Cook the meal for 15 minutes.

Nutrition:

Calories: 147;

Protein: 4.3g;

Carbs: 4.1g;

Fat: 5.9g

Bulgur Bowl

Preparation Time: 10 minutes

Cooking Time: 0 minutes

Servings: 4

Ingredients:

- 6 oz salmon, boiled, chopped
- ½ cup bulgur, cooked
- 1 cup fresh cilantro, chopped
- 1 cup tomato, chopped
- 3 tbsp. lemon juice
- 1 tbsp. olive oil

Directions:

1. Put salmon, bulgur, cilantro, and tomato in the bowl.
2. Add lemon juice and olive oil.
3. Shake the mixture well and transfer in the serving bowls.

Nutrition:

Calories: 153;

Protein: 12.3g;

Carbs: 6.4g;

Fat: 11.4g

Boiled Bulgur with Kale

Preparation Time: 10 minutes

Cooking Time: 11 minutes

Servings: 6

Ingredients:

- 1 cup bulgur
- cups water
- 1 cup kale
- ½ zucchini, chopped
- ½ tsp. allspices
- 6 tbsp. olive oil
- 2 oz goat cheese, crumbled

Directions:

1. Mix water and bulgur in the saucepan and cook boil for 11 minutes.
2. Then cool the bulgur and mix it with chopped kale, zucchini, allspices, and olive oil.
3. Transfer the bulgur meal in the serving bowls and top with goat cheese.

Nutrition:

Calories: 251;

Protein: 6.3g;

Carbs: 3.4g;

Fat: 6.3g

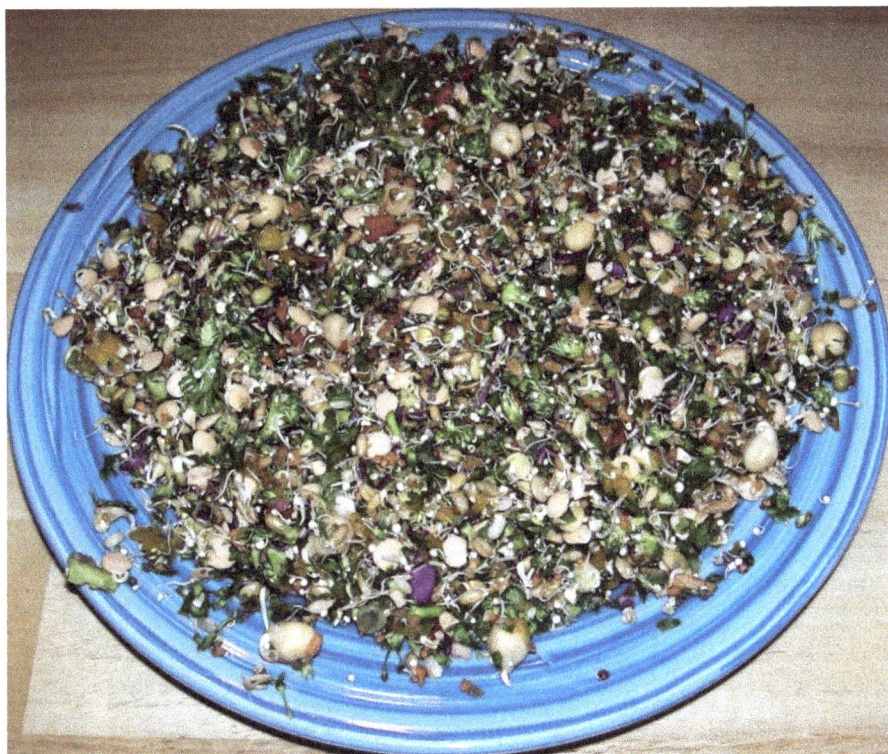

Chicken and Rice Soup

Preparation Time: 10 minutes

Cooking Time: 20 minutes

Servings: 6

Ingredients:

- 4 cups chicken stock
- 1 cup of water
- 1-lb. chicken breast, shredded
- 1 cup of rice, cooked
- 3 egg yolks
- 3 tbsp. lemon juice
- 1/3 cup fresh parsley, chopped
- ½ tsp. salt
- ¼ tsp. ground black pepper

Directions:

1. Pour water and chicken stock in the saucepan and bring to boil.
2. Then pour one cup of the hot liquid in the food processor.

3. Add cooked rice, egg yolks, lemon juice, and salt. Blend the mixture until smooth.
4. After this, transfer the smooth rice mixture into the saucepan with remaining chicken stock liquid.
5. Add shredded chicken breast, parsley, and ground black pepper.
6. Boil the soup for 5 minutes more.

Nutrition:

Calories 235,

Fat 4.8,

Carbs 25.9,

Protein 20.2

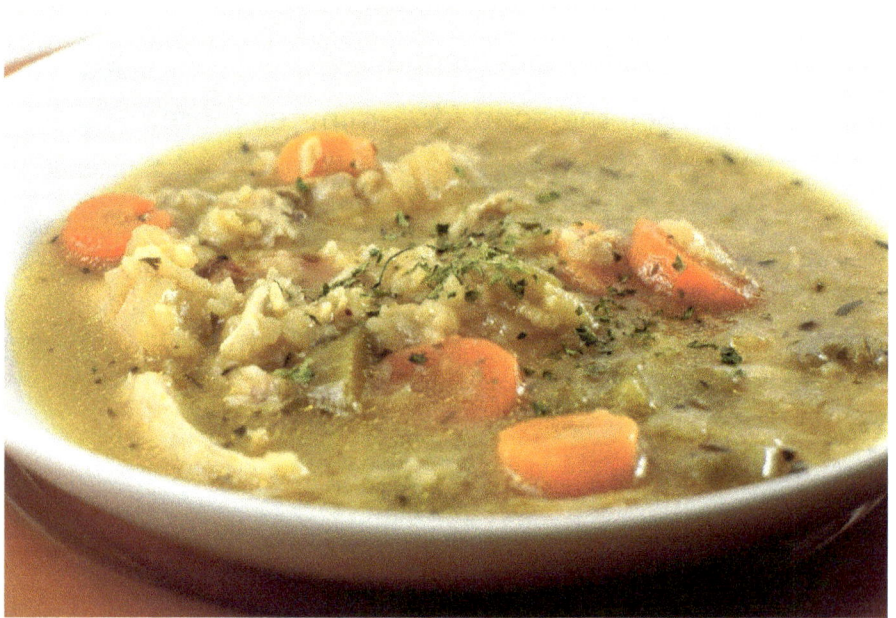

Tomato Bulgur

Preparation Time: 5 minutes

Cooking Time: 20 minutes

Servings: 3

Ingredients:

- ½ cup bulgur
- 1 onion, diced
- 3 tbsp. tomato paste
- ½ tsp. salt
- 2 tbsp. olive oil
- 1 cup of water

Directions:

1. Melt the olive oil in the saucepan.
2. Add diced onion and cook it until light brown.
3. Then add bulgur and tomato paste. Stir the ingredients.
4. Add water and cook the meal for 15 minutes.

Nutrition: 186 Calories, 4g Protein, 24.2g Carbs, 9.5g Fat

Bulgur Mix

Preparation Time: 10 minutes

Cooking Time: 0 minutes

Servings: 3

Ingredients:

- ½ cup bulgur, cooked
- ¼ cup corn kernels, cooked
- ¼ cup chickpeas, cooked
- ¼ cup snap peas, cooked
- 4 tbsp. plain yogurt

Directions:

1. Put all ingredients in the big bowl and carefully stir.

Nutrition: 176 Calories, 8.3g Protein, 33.4g Carbs, 1.8g Fat

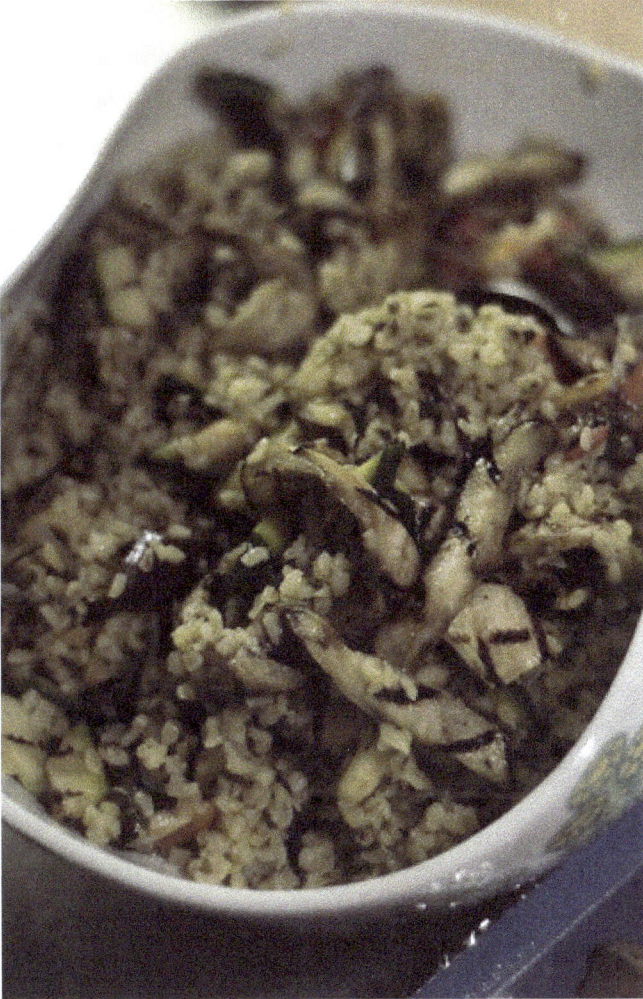

Aromatic Baked Brown Rice

Preparation Time: 10 minutes

Cooking Time: 20 minutes

Servings: 6

Ingredients:

- ½ cup minced fresh parsley
- ¾ cup jarred roasted red peppers, rinsed, patted dry, and chopped
- 1 cup chicken or vegetable broth
- 1½ cups long-grain brown rice, rinsed
- 2 onions, chopped fine
- 2¼ cups water
- 4 tsp. extra-virgin olive oil
- Grated Parmesan cheese
- Lemon wedges
- Salt and pepper

Directions:

1. Place the oven rack in the centre of the oven and pre-heat your oven to 375°F. Heat oil in a Dutch oven on moderate heat until it starts to

shimmer. Put in onions and 1 tsp. salt and cook, stirring intermittently, till they become tender and well browned, 12 to 14 minutes.

2.   Mix in water and broth and bring to boil. Mix in rice, cover, and move pot to oven. Bake until rice becomes soft and liquid is absorbed, 65 to 70 minutes.

3.   Remove pot from oven. Sprinkle red peppers over rice, cover, and allow to sit for about five minutes. Put in parsley to rice and fluff gently with fork to combine. Sprinkle with salt and pepper to taste. Serve with grated Parmesan and lemon wedges.

Nutrition:

Calories: 302

Protein: 8 g

Fat: 14 g

Carbs: 23 g

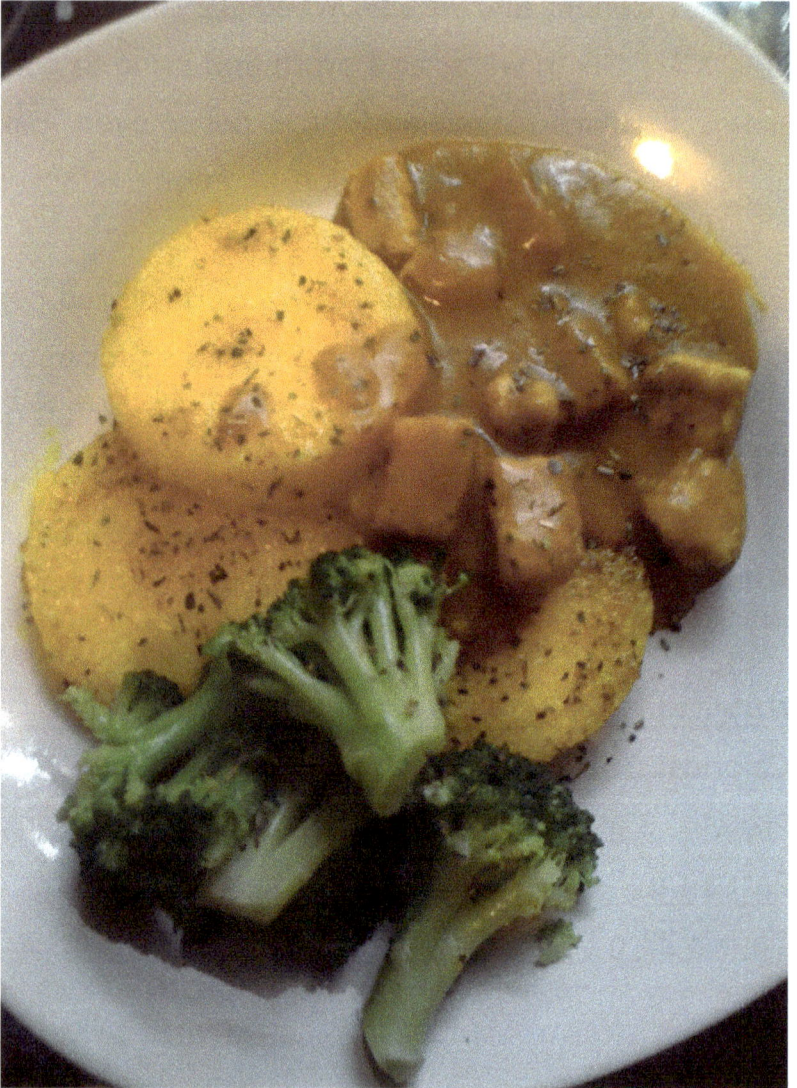

Aromatic Barley Pilaf

Preparation Time: 10 minutes

Cooking Time: 10 minutes

Servings: 6

Ingredients:

- ¼ cup minced fresh parsley
- 1 small onion, chopped fine
- 1½ cups pearl barley, rinsed
- 1½ tsp. lemon juice
- 1½ tsp. minced fresh thyme or ½ tsp. dried
- 2 garlic cloves, minced
- 2 tbsp. minced fresh chives
- 2½ cups water
- 3 tbsp. extra-virgin olive oil
- Salt and pepper

Directions:

1. Heat oil in a big saucepan on moderate heat until it starts to shimmer. Put in onion and ½ tsp. salt and cook till they become tender, approximately five minutes. Mix in barley, garlic, and thyme and cook, stirring often, until barley is lightly toasted and aromatic, approximately three minutes.

2. Mix in water and bring to simmer. Decrease heat to low, cover, and simmer until barley becomes soft and water is absorbed, 20 to 40 minutes.

3. Remove from the heat, lay clean dish towel underneath lid and let pilaf sit for about ten minutes. Put in parsley, chives, and lemon juice to pilaf and fluff gently with fork to combine. Sprinkle with salt and pepper to taste. Serve.

Nutrition:

Calories: 222

Protein: 18 g

Fat: 14 g

Carbs: 22 g

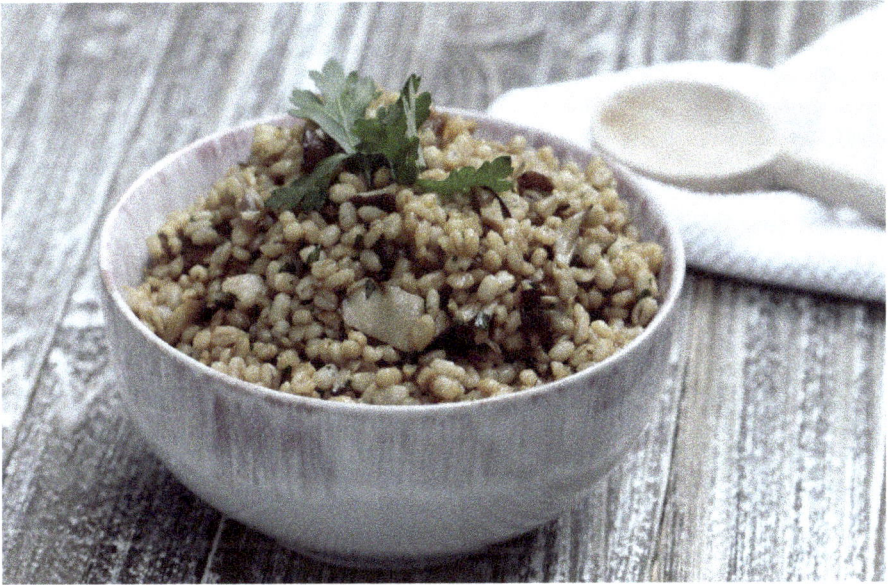

Basmati Rice Pilaf Mix

Preparation Time: 10 minutes

Cooking Time: 15 minutes

Servings:

Ingredients:

- ¼ cup currants
- ¼ cup sliced almonds, toasted
- ¼ tsp. ground cinnamon
- ½ tsp. ground turmeric
- 1 small onion, chopped fine
- 1 tbsp. extra-virgin olive oil
- 1½ cups basmati rice, rinsed
- 2 garlic cloves, minced
- 2¼ cups water
- Salt and pepper

Directions:

1. Heat oil in a big saucepan on moderate heat until it starts to shimmer. Put in onion and ¼ tsp. salt and cook till they become tender, approximately five minutes. Put in rice, garlic,

turmeric, and cinnamon and cook, stirring often, until grain edges begin to turn translucent, approximately three minutes.

2.   Mix in water and bring to simmer. Decrease heat to low, cover, and simmer gently until rice becomes soft and water is absorbed, 16 to 18 minutes.

3.   Remove from the heat, drizzle currants over pilaf. Cover, laying clean dish towel underneath lid, and let pilaf sit for about ten minutes. Put in almonds to pilaf and fluff gently with fork to combine. Sprinkle with salt and pepper to taste. Serve.

Nutrition:

Calories: 234

Protein: 8 g

Fat: 11 g

Carbs: 33 g

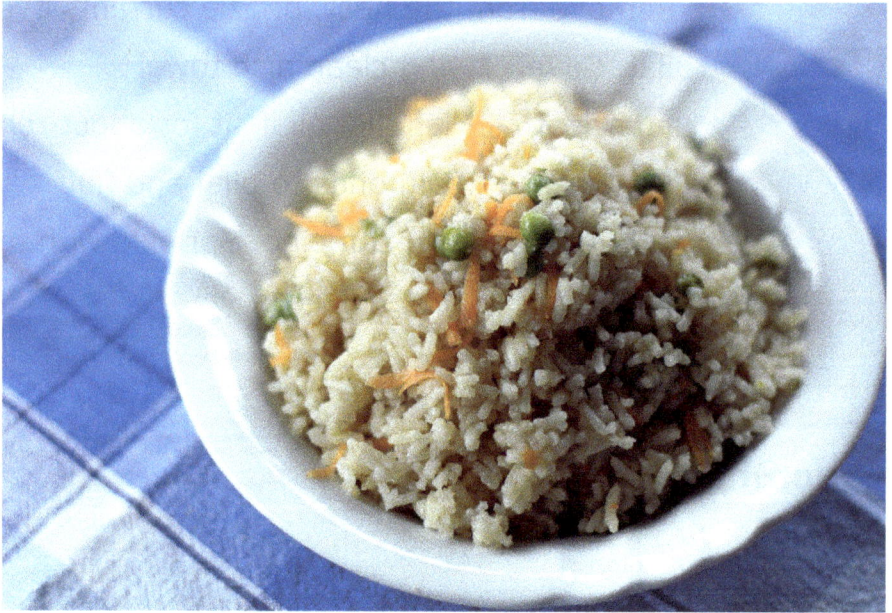

Brown Rice Salad with Asparagus, Goat Cheese, and Lemon

Preparation Time: 10 minutes

Cooking Time: 15 minutes

Servings: 2

Ingredients:

- ¼ cup minced fresh parsley
- ¼ cup slivered almonds, toasted
- 1 lb. asparagus, trimmed and cut into 1-inch lengths
- 1 shallot, minced
- 1 tsp. grated lemon zest plus 3 tbsp. juice
- 1½ cups long-grain brown rice
- 2 oz. goat cheese, crumbled (½ cup)
- 3½ tbsp. extra-virgin olive oil
- Salt and pepper

Directions:

1. Bring 4 quarts water to boil in a Dutch oven. Put in rice and 1½ tsp. salt and cook, stirring intermittently, until rice is tender, about half an hour. Drain rice, spread onto rimmed baking sheet, and drizzle with 1 tbsp. lemon juice. Allow it to cool completely, about fifteen minutes.

2. Heat 1 tbsp. oil in 12-inch frying pan on high heat until just smoking. Put in asparagus, ¼ tsp. salt, and ¼ tsp. pepper and cook, stirring intermittently, until asparagus is browned and crisp-tender, about 4 minutes; move to plate and allow to cool slightly.
3. Beat remaining 2½ tbsp. oil, lemon zest and remaining 2 tbsp. juice, shallot, ½ tsp. salt, and ½ tsp. pepper together in a big container.
4. Put in rice, asparagus, 2 tbsp. goat cheese, 3 tbsp. almonds, and 3 tbsp. parsley. Gently toss to combine and allow to sit for about ten minutes. Sprinkle with salt and pepper to taste.
5. Move to serving platter and drizzle with remaining 2 tbsp. goat cheese, remaining 1 tbsp. almonds, and remaining 1 tbsp. parsley. Serve.

Nutrition:

Calories: 242

Protein: 18 g

Fat: 8 g

Carbs: 12 g

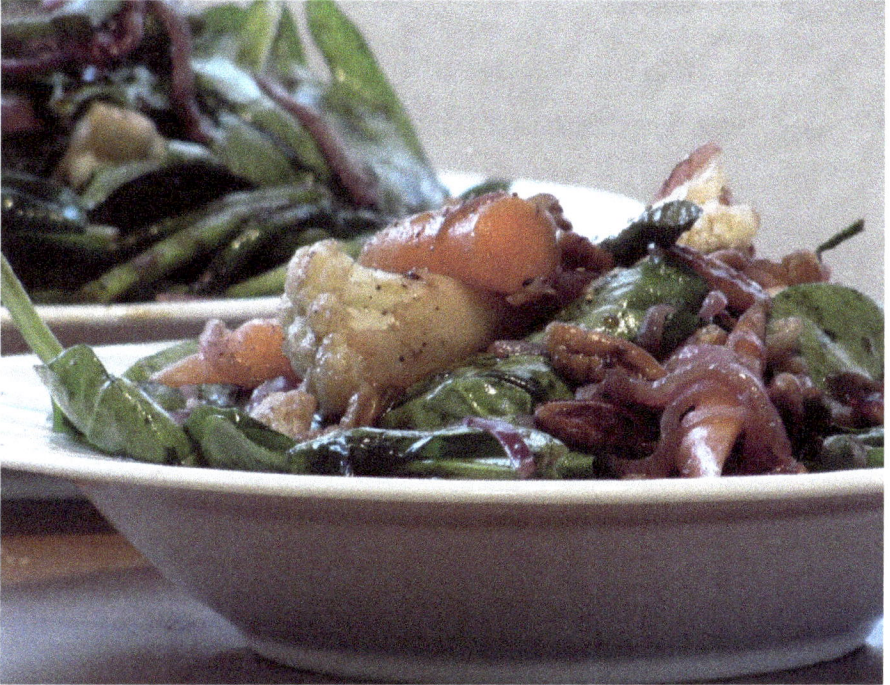

Carrot-Almond-Bulgur Salad

Preparation Time: 10 minutes

Cooking Time: 20 minutes

Servings: 4

Ingredients:

- 1/8 tsp. cayenne pepper
- 1/3 cup chopped fresh cilantro
- 1/3 cup chopped fresh mint
- 1/3 cup extra-virgin olive oil
- ½ cup sliced almonds, toasted
- ½ tsp. ground cumin
- 1 cup water
- 1½ cups medium-grind bulgur, rinsed
- 3 scallions, sliced thin
- 4 carrots, peeled and shredded
- 6 tbsp. lemon juice (2 lemons)
- Salt and pepper

Directions:

1. Mix bulgur, water, ¼ cup lemon juice, and ¼ tsp. salt in a container. Cover and allow to sit at room temperature until grains are softened and liquid is fully absorbed, about 1½ hours.
2. Beat remaining 2 tbsp. lemon juice, oil, cumin, cayenne, and ½ tsp. salt together in a big container.
3. Put in bulgur, carrots, scallions, almonds, mint, and cilantro and gently toss to combine. Sprinkle with salt and pepper to taste. Serve.

Nutrition:

Calories: 287

Protein: 8 g

Fat: 7 g

Carbs: 13 g

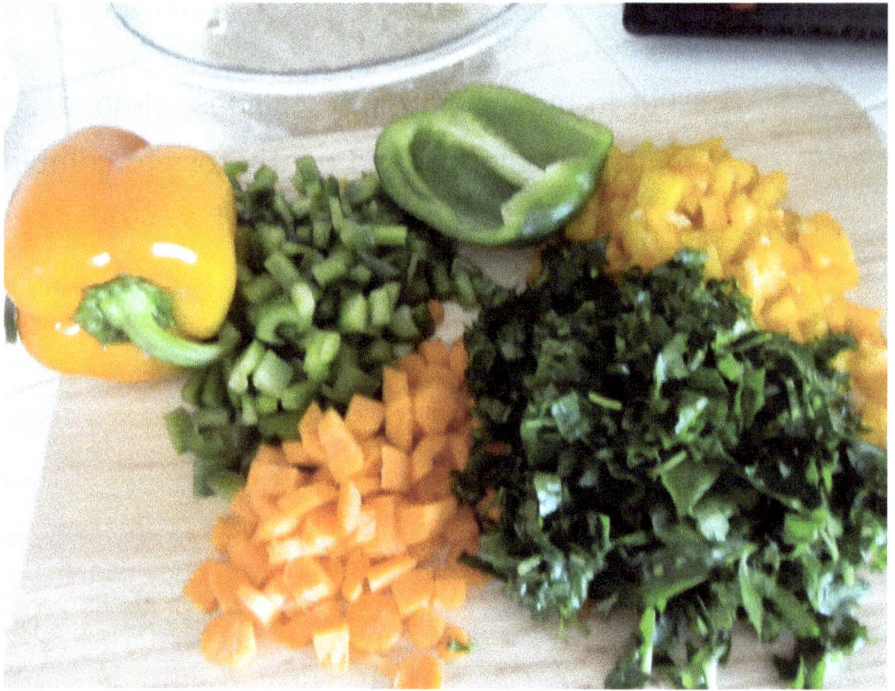

Chickpea-Spinach Bulgur

Preparation Time: 5 minutes

Cooking Time: 20 minutes

Servings: 6

Ingredients:

- ¾ cup chicken or vegetable broth
- ¾ cup water
- 1 (15-oz.) can chickpeas, rinsed
- 1 cup medium-grind bulgur, rinsed
- 1 onion, chopped fine
- 1 tbsp. lemon juice
- 2 tbsp. za'atar
- 3 garlic cloves, minced
- 3 oz. (3 cups) baby spinach, chopped
- 3 tbsp. extra-virgin olive oil
- Salt and pepper

Directions:

1. Heat 2 tbsp. oil in a big saucepan on moderate heat until it starts to shimmer. Put

in onion and ½ tsp. salt and cook till they become tender, approximately five minutes. Mix in garlic and 1 tbsp. za'atar and cook until aromatic, approximately half a minute.

2.   Mix in bulgur, chickpeas, broth, and water and bring to simmer. Decrease heat to low, cover, and simmer gently until bulgur is tender, 16 to 18 minutes.

3.   Remove from the heat, lay clean dish towel underneath lid and let bulgur sit for about ten minutes. Put in spinach, lemon juice, remaining 1 tbsp. za'atar, and residual 1 tbsp. oil and fluff gently with fork to combine. Sprinkle with salt and pepper to taste. Serve.

Nutrition:

Calories: 234

Protein: 18 g

Fat: 14 g

Carbs: 10 g

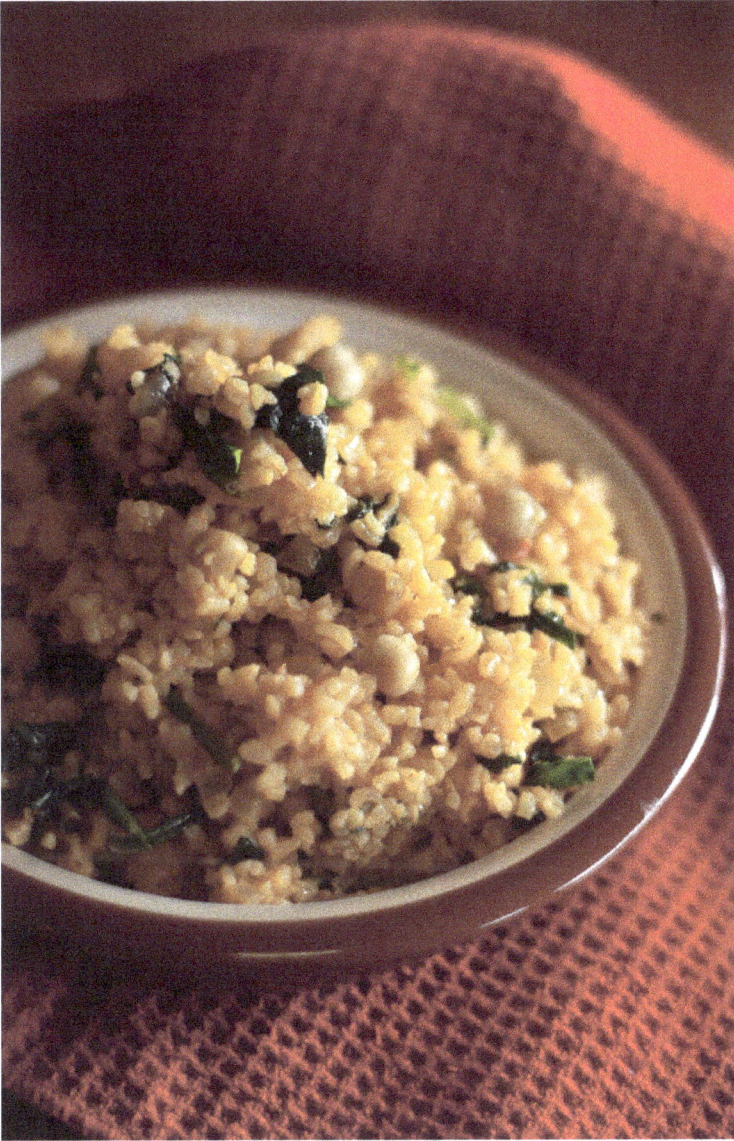

Classic Baked Brown Rice

Preparation Time: 10 minutes

Cooking Time: 20 minutes

Servings: 6

Ingredients:

- 1½ cups long-grain brown rice, rinsed
- 2 tsp. extra-virgin olive oil
- 2 1/3 cups boiling water
- Salt and pepper

Directions:

1. Place the oven rack in the centre of the oven and pre-heat your oven to 375°F. Mix boiling water, rice, oil, and ½ tsp. salt in 8-inch square baking dish.

2. Cover dish tightly using double layer of aluminium foil. Bake until rice becomes soft and water is absorbed, about 1 hour. Remove

dish from oven, uncover, and gently fluff rice with fork, scraping up any rice that has stuck to bottom.

3.   Cover dish with clean dish towel and let rice sit for about five minutes. Uncover and let rice sit for about five minutes longer.

4.   Sprinkle with salt and pepper to taste. Serve.

Nutrition:

Calories: 222

Protein: 18 g

Fat: 10 g

Carbs: 12 g

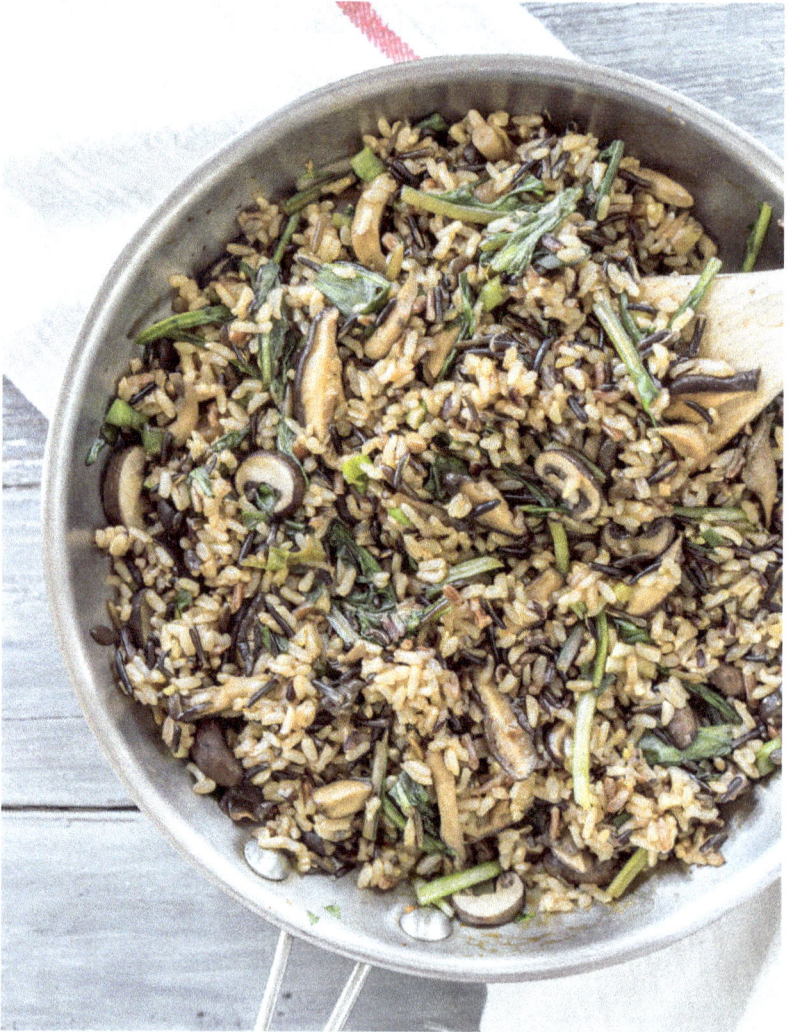

Classic Italian Seafood Risotto

Preparation Time: 10 minutes

Cooking Time: 20 minutes

Servings: 4

Ingredients:

- 1/8 tsp. saffron threads, crumbled
- 1 (14.5-oz.) can diced tomatoes, drained
- 1 cup dry white wine
- 1 onion, chopped fine
- 1 tbsp. lemon juice
- 1 tsp. minced fresh thyme or ¼ tsp. dried
- 12 oz. large shrimp (26 to 30 per lb.), peeled and deveined, shells reserved
- 12 oz. small bay scallops
- 2 bay leaves
- 2 cups Arborio rice
- 2 cups chicken broth
- 2 tbsp. minced fresh parsley
- 2½ cups water
- 4 (8-oz.) bottles clam juice
- 5 garlic cloves, minced
- 5 tbsp. extra-virgin olive oil
- Salt and pepper

Directions:

1. Bring shrimp shells, broth, water, clam juice, tomatoes, and bay leaves to boil in a big saucepan on moderate to high heat.

2. Decrease the heat to a simmer and cook for 20 minutes. Strain mixture through fine-mesh strainer into big container, pressing on solids to extract as much liquid as possible; discard solids. Return broth to now-empty saucepan, cover, and keep warm on low heat.

3. Heat 2 tbsp. oil in a Dutch oven on moderate heat until it starts to shimmer. Put in onion and cook till they become tender, approximately five minutes.

4. Put in rice, garlic, thyme, and saffron and cook, stirring often, until grain edges begin to turn translucent, approximately three minutes.

5. Put in wine and cook, stirring often, until fully absorbed, approximately three minutes. Mix in 3½ cups warm broth, bring to simmer, and cook, stirring intermittently, until almost fully absorbed, about fifteen minutes.

6. Carry on cooking rice, stirring often and adding warm broth, 1 cup at a time, every few minutes as liquid is absorbed, until rice is

creamy and cooked through but still somewhat firm in center, about fifteen minutes.

7. Mix in shrimp and scallops and cook, stirring often, until opaque throughout, approximately three minutes. Remove pot from heat, cover, and allow to sit for about five minutes.

8. Adjust consistency with remaining warm broth as required (you may have broth left over). Mix in remaining 3 tbsp. oil, parsley, and lemon juice and sprinkle with salt and pepper to taste. Serve.

Nutrition:

Calories: 343

Protein: 18 g

Fat: 14 g

Carbs: 33 g

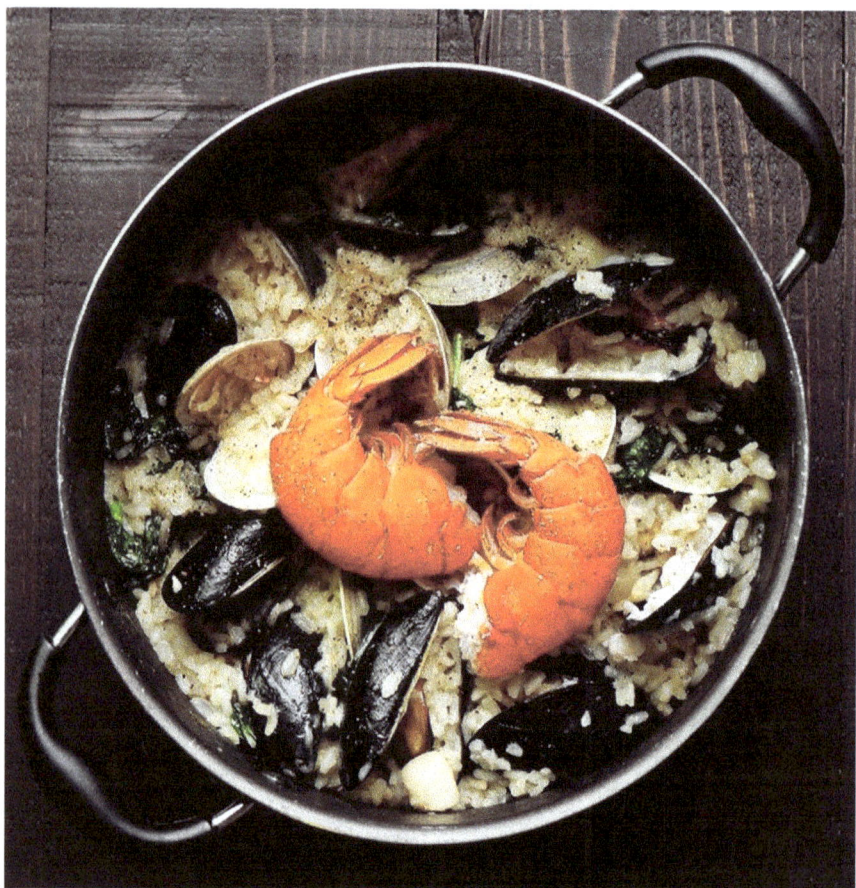

Classic Stovetop White Rice

Preparation Time: 10 minutes

Cooking Time: 10 minutes

Servings: 6

Ingredients:

- 1 tbsp. extra-virgin olive oil
- 2 cups long-grain white rice, rinsed
- 3 cups water
- Basmati, jasmine, or Texmati rice can be substituted for the long-grain rice.
- Salt and pepper

Directions:

1. Heat oil in a big saucepan on moderate heat until it starts to shimmer. Put in rice and cook, stirring frequently, until grain edges begin to turn translucent, approximately two minutes.

2. Put in water and 1 tsp. salt and bring to simmer. Cover, decrease the heat to low, and simmer gently until rice becomes soft and water is absorbed, approximately twenty minutes.

3. Remove from the heat, lay clean dish towel underneath lid and let rice sit for about ten minutes. Gently fluff rice with fork. Sprinkle with salt and pepper to taste. Serve.

Nutrition:

Calories: 252

Protein: 18 g

Fat: 10 g

Carbs: 33 g

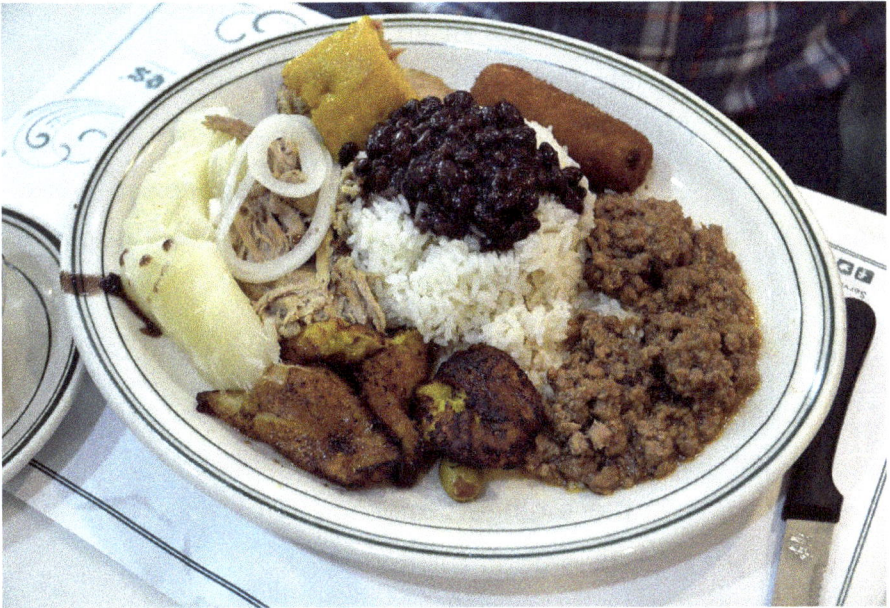

Moroccan Lentil Soup

Preparation Time: 10 minutes

Cooking Time: 1 hour

Servings: 6

Ingredients:

- 2 tbsp. extra virgin olive oil
- 1 large yellow onion, finely chopped
- 2 stalks celery, finely chopped
- 1 carrot, peeled and finely chopped
- 1/3 cup chopped parsley, leaves and tender stems
- 1/2 cup chopped cilantro, leaves and tender stems
- 5 large garlic cloves, minced
- 2" piece ginger, minced
- 1 tsp. ground turmeric
- 1 tsp. ground cinnamon
- 2 tsp. sweet paprika
- 1/2 tsp. Aleppo pepper (or substitute freshly ground black pepper)
- 1 1/4 cups dry red lentils, rinsed and picked over
- 1 x 15 oz. can garbanzo beans, drained
- 1 x 28 oz. can sieved tomatoes
- 7–8 cups chicken broth or vegetable broth

- Coarse salt

To Servings:

- Dates
- Lemon wedges

Directions:

1. Grab a large saucepan, add the olive oil and place over a medium heat.
2. Add the onion, celery, carrots, garlic, and ginger and cook for 5 minutes until soft.
3. Throw in the turmeric, cinnamon, paprika and pepper and continue to cook for another 5 minutes.
4. Add the tomatoes and broth, stir well then bring to a simmer.
5. Add the lentils, garbanzo beans, cilantro and parsley.
6. Cook uncovered for 35 minutes until the lentils become very soft.
7. Season well then serve and enjoy.

Nutrition:

Calories: 551;

Protein: 36.3g;

Carbs: 33.4g;

Fat: 30.3g

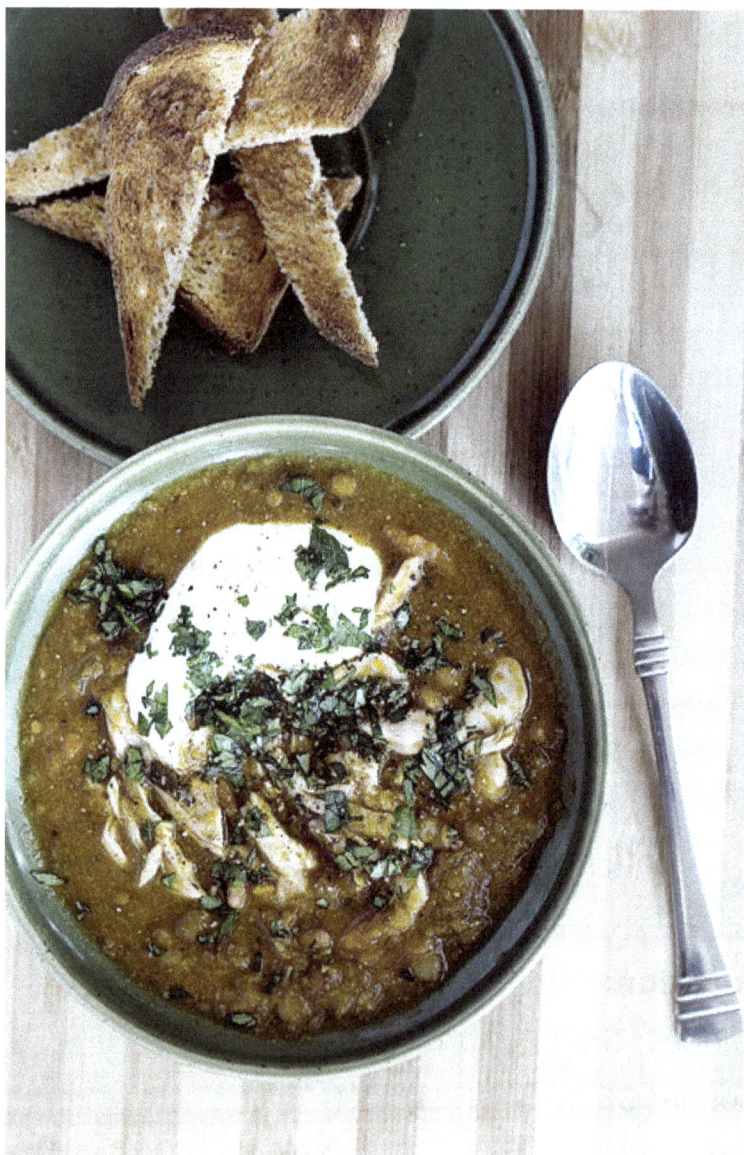

Roasted Red Pepper and Tomato Soup

Preparation Time: 10 minutes

Cooking Time: 45 minutes

Servings: 4

Ingredients:

- 2 red bell peppers, seeded and halved
- 3 tomatoes, cored and halved
- 1/2 medium onion, quartered
- 2 cloves garlic, peeled and halved
- 1-2 tbsp. olive oil
- 1/4 tsp. salt
- 1/4 tsp. ground black pepper
- 2 cups vegetable broth
- 2 tbsp. tomato paste
- 1/4 cup fresh parsley, chopped
- 1/4 tsp. Italian seasoning blend
- 1/4 tsp. ground paprika
- 1/8 teaspoon. ground cayenne pepper, or more to taste

Directions:

1. Preheat your oven to 375°F.
2. Grab a medium bowl and add the red peppers, tomatoes, onion, garlic, olive oil and salt and pepper. Toss well to coat.

3. Place onto a baking sheet and pop into the oven for 45 minutes until soft.
4. Next place the veggie broth over a medium heat and add the roasted veggies, tomato paste, parsley, paprika and cayenne.
5. Stir to combine then simmer for 10 minutes.
6. Use an immersion blender to puree the soup then return back to the pan.
7. Reheat if required, add extra seasoning then serve and enjoy.

Nutrition:

Calories: 531;

Protein: 26.3g;

Carbs: 33.4g;

Fat: 30.3g

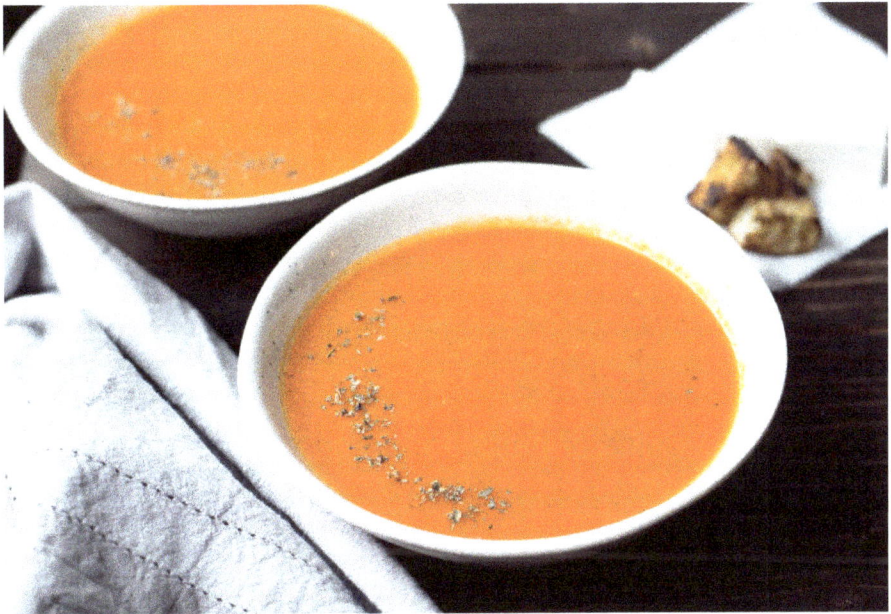

Greek Spring Soup

Preparation Time: 10 minutes

Cooking Time: 35 minutes

Servings: 4

Ingredients:

- 6 cups chicken broth
- 1 1/2 cups diced or shredded cooked chicken
- 2 tbsp. olive oil
- 1 small onion, diced
- 1 bay leaf
- 1/3 cup arborio rice
- 1 large free-range egg
- 2 tbsp. water
- Juice of half of a lemon
- 1 cup chopped asparagus
- 1 cup diced carrots
- 1/2 cup fresh chopped dill, divided
- Salt and pepper, to taste

Directions:

1. Find a large pan, add the oil and place over a medium heat.
2. Add the onions and cook for five minutes until soft.

3. Next add ¼ cup dill, plus the chicken broth and bay leaf. Bring to a boil.
4. Add the rice and reduce the heat to low. Simmer for 10 minutes.
5. Add the carrots and asparagus and cook for 10 more minutes until the rice and veggies are tender.
6. Add the chicken and simmer.
7. Meanwhile find a medium bowl and add the egg, lemon and water. Whisk well.
8. Add ½ cup of the stock to the egg mixture, stirring constantly then pour it all back into the pot.
9. Heat through and allow the soup to thicken.
10. Add remaining dill, season well then serve and enjoy.

Nutrition:

Calories: 551;

Protein: 16.3g;

Carbs: 23.4g;

Fat: 10.3g

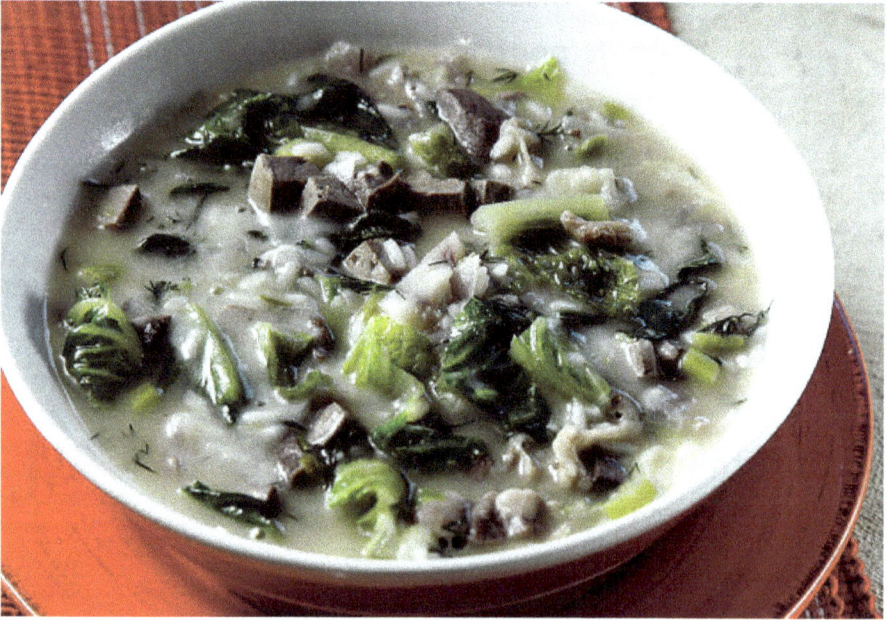

Fast Seafood Gumbo

Preparation Time: 10 minutes

Cooking Time: 40 minutes

Servings: 4

Ingredients:

- 1/4 cup olive oil
- 1/4 cup flour
- 1 medium white onion, chopped
- 1 cup celery, chopped
- 1 red or green bell pepper, chopped and deseeded
- 1 red chili, chopped
- 2 cups okra, chopped
- 1 cup canned crushed tomatoes
- 2 large cloves garlic, crushed
- 1 tsp. dried thyme
- 2 cups fish stock
- 1 bay leaf
- 1 tsp. cayenne powder
- 2 x 8 oz. can crab meat with brine
- 1 lb. shrimp, peeled and deveined
- Salt & pepper, to taste
- 1/4 cup fresh parsley, finely chopped

Directions:

1. Find a large pan, add the oil and place over a medium heat.
2. Add the flour and stir well until it forms a thick paste.
3. Add the onions, celery, peppers and okra and stir well, cooking for 5 minutes.
4. Add the garlic, tomatoes, thyme, stock, bay leaf and cayenne and stir again.
5. Bring to a boil then reduce the heat and simmer for 15 minutes.
6. Add the shrimp and crab and cook for 8 minutes more.

Nutrition:

Calories: 551;

Protein: 36.3g;

Carbs: 33.4g;

Fat: 30.3g

Minestrone Soup

Preparation Time: 10 minutes

Cooking Time: 1 hour

Servings: 4

Ingredients:

- 1 small white onion, minced
- 4 cloves garlic, minced
- 1/2 cup sliced carrots
- 1 medium zucchini sliced, then cut slices in half
- 1 medium yellow squash sliced, then cut slices in half
- 2 tbsp. minced fresh parsley
- 1/4 cup celery sliced
- 3 tbsp. olive oil
- 2 x 15 oz. cans cannellini beans, rinsed & drained
- 2 x 15 oz. cans red kidney beans, rinsed & drained

- 1 x 14.5 oz. can fire-roasted diced tomatoes, drained
- 4 cups vegetable stock
- 2 cups water
- 1 1/2 tsp. oregano
- 1/2 tsp. basil
- 1/4 tsp. thyme
- 1 tsp. salt
- 1/2 tsp. pepper
- 3/4 cup small pasta shells
- 4 cups fresh baby spinach
- 1/4 cup Parmesan or Romano cheese

Directions:

1. Grab a stock pot and place over a medium heat.
2. Add the oil then the onions, garlic, carrots, zucchini, squash, parsley and celery.
3. Cook for five minutes until the veggies are getting soft.
4. Pour in the stock, water, beans, tomatoes, herbs and salt and pepper. Stir well.

5. Reduce the heat, cover and simmer for 30 minutes.
6. Add the pasta and spinach, stir well then cover and cook for a further 20 minutes until the pasta is cooked through.
7. Stir through the cheese then serve and enjoy.

Nutrition:

Calories 34;

Protein: 26.3g;

Carbs: 33.4g;

Fat: 30.3g

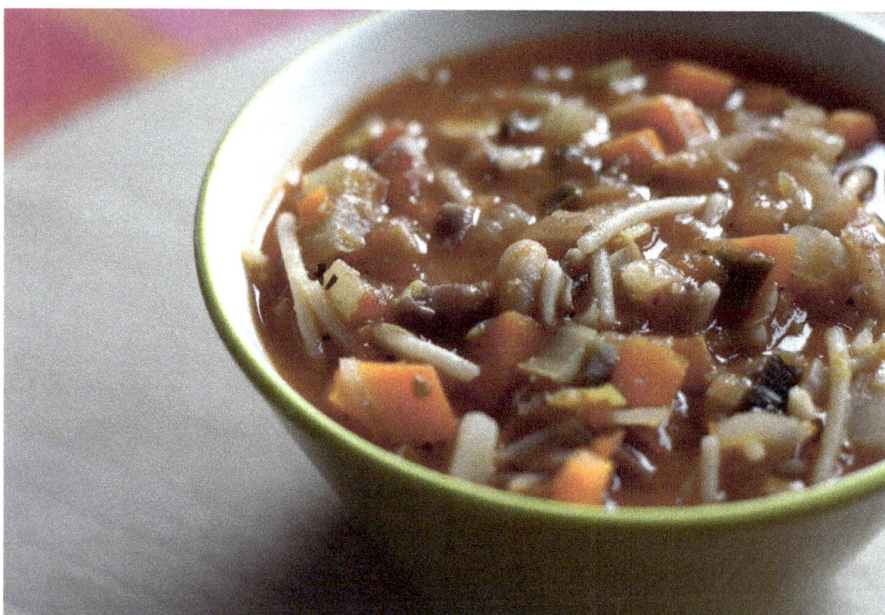

Lemon Chicken Soup

Preparation Time: 10 minutes

Cooking Time: 20 minutes

Servings: 6

Ingredients:

- 10 cups chicken broth
- 3 tbsp. olive oil
- 8 cloves garlic, minced
- 1 sweet onion, sliced
- 1 large lemon, zested
- 2 boneless skinless chicken breasts
- 1 cup Israeli couscous
- 1/2 tsp. crushed red pepper
- 2 oz. crumbled feta
- 1/3 cup chopped chive
- Salt and pepper, to taste

Directions:

1. Grab a stock pot, add the oil and place over a medium heat.
2. Add the onion and garlic and cook for five minutes until soft.
3. Add the broth, chicken breasts, lemon zest and crushed pepper.

4. Raise the heat, cover and bring to a boil.

5.   Reduce the heat then simmer for 5 minutes.

6. Turn off the heat, remove the lid and remove the chicken from the pot.

7. Pop onto a place and use two forks to shred.

8. Pop back into the pot, add the feta, chives and salt and pepper.

9. Stir well then serve and enjoy.

Nutrition:

Calories: 251;

Protein: 16.3g;

Carbs: 23.4g;

Fat: 30.3g

Tuscan Vegetable Pasta Soup

Preparation Time: 10 minutes

Cooking Time: 30 minutes

Servings: 6

Ingredients:

- 2 tbsp. extra virgin olive oil
- 4 cloves garlic, minced
- 1 medium yellow onion, diced
- 1/2 cup carrot, chopped
- 1/2 cup celery, chopped
- 1 medium zucchini, sliced and quartered
- 1 x 15 oz. can diced tomatoes
- 6 cups vegetable stock
- 2 tbsp. tomato paste
- 6-8 oz. whole wheat pasta
- 1 x 15 oz. can white beans
- 2 large handfuls baby spinach
- 6 basil cubes
- Salt and pepper, to taste
- Fresh chopped parsley, for garnish

Directions:

1. Grab a stock pot, add the oil and pop over a medium heat.
2. Add the onion and garlic and cook for five minutes until soft.

3. Throw in the carrots, celery and zucchini and cook for an extra 5 minutes, stirring occasionally.
4. Add the tomato and salt and pepper and cook for 1-2 minutes.
5. Add the veggies broth and tomato paste, stir well then bring to the boil.
6. Throw in the pasta, cook for 10 minutes then add the spinach, white beans, basil cubes and seasoning.
7. Stir well then remove from the heat.
8. Divide between large bowls and serve and enjoy.

Nutrition:

Calories: 151;

Protein: 26.3g;

Carbs: 14.4g;

Fat: 30.3g

Dairy Free Zucchini Soup

Preparation Time: 10 minutes

Cooking Time: 25 minutes

Servings: 8

Ingredients:

- 2½ lb. zucchini
- 1 medium onion, diced
- 2 tbsp. olive oil
- 4 garlic cloves, chopped
- 4 cups chicken stock
- Sea salt and pepper, to taste
- 1/3 cup fresh basil leaves

Directions:

1. Grab a pan, add the oil and pop over a medium heat.
2. Add the onion, garlic and zucchini and cook for five minutes until soft.
3. Add the stock and simmer for 15 minutes.

4. Remove from the heat, stir through the basil, add the seasoning and use an immersion blender to whizz until smooth.
5. Serve and enjoy.

Nutrition:

Calories: 551;

Protein: 36.3g;

Carbs: 33.4g;

Fat: 30.3g

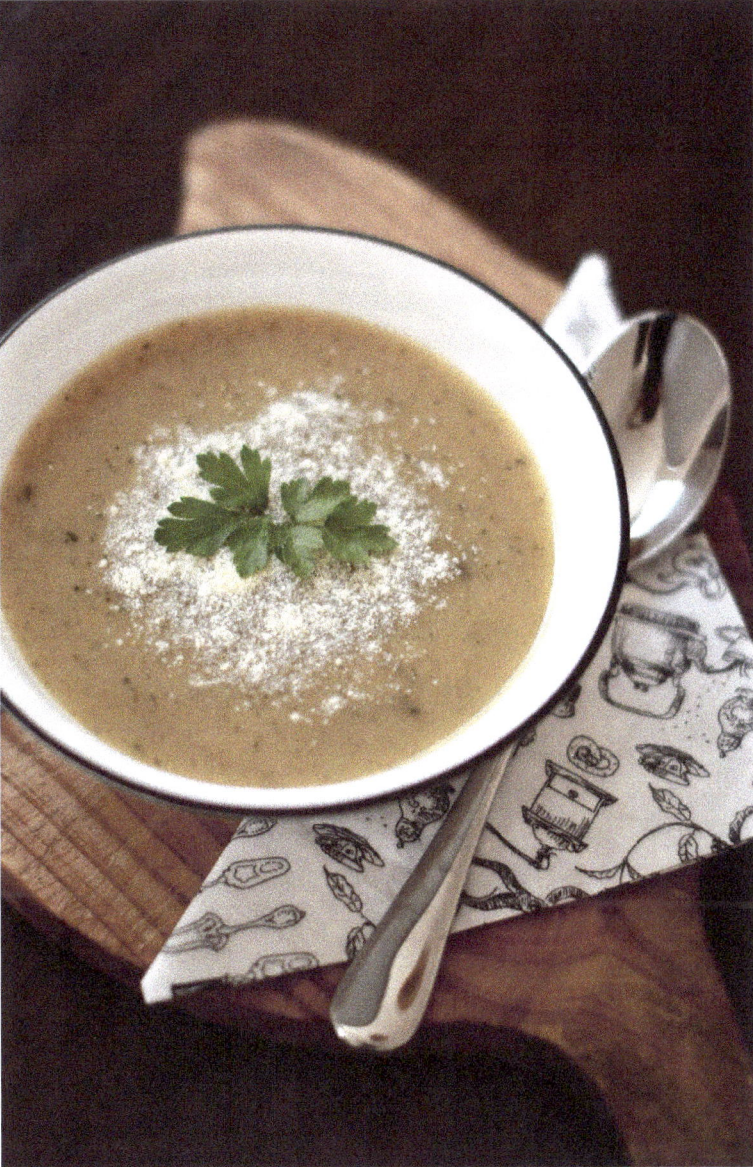

Farro Stew with Kale & Cannellini Beans

Preparation Time: 10 minutes

Cooking Time 1 hour

Servings: 4

Ingredients:

- 2 tbsp. olive oil
- 2 medium carrots, diced
- 1 medium onion, chopped
- 2 sticks celery, chopped
- 4 cloves garlic, minced
- 5 cups low-sodium vegetable broth
- 1 x 14.5 oz. can diced tomatoes
- 1 cup farro, rinsed
- 1 tsp. dried oregano
- 1 bay leaf
- Salt, to taste
- 1/2 cup parsley
- 4 cups chopped kale, thick ribs removed
- 1 x 15 oz. can cannellini beans, drained and rinsed
- 1 tbsp. fresh lemon juice
- 1/2 cup feta cheese, crumbled

Directions:

1. Grab a stock pot, add the oil and place over a medium heat.
2. Add the onion, carrots and celery and cook for five minutes until becoming soft.
3. Add the garlic and cook for another 30 seconds.
4. Stir through the broth, tomatoes, farro, oregano, bay leaf, parsley and salt.
5. Cover with the lid and bring to the boil. Reduce the heat then simmer for 20 minutes.
6. Remove the lid, add the kale and cook for a further 10-15 minutes.
7. Remove the bay leaf, add the beans, stir through the lemon juice and any additional liquid then stir well to combine.
8. Serve and enjoy.

Nutrition:

Calories: 21;

Protein: 16.3g;

Carbs: 3.4g;

Fat: 6.3g

Italian Meatball Soup

Preparation Time: 10 minutes

Cooking Time: 45 minutes

Servings: 6

Ingredients:

- 1/4 - 1/2 cup freshly grated parmesan cheese (optional)
- 1 free-range egg
- 1 cup breadcrumbs, optional
- 2 tbsp. fresh parsley, minced
- 1 tsp. dried oregano
- 1/2 tsp. sea salt
- ½ tsp. black pepper
- 3 tbsp. olive oil

For the soup...

- 2 quarts chicken broth or beef broth
- 3 tbsp. tomato paste
- 1 onion, diced
- 2 bay leaves
- 4-5 sprigs fresh thyme
- ½ tsp. whole black peppercorns

To serve...

- Fresh parmesan cheese, grated
- 1-2 tbsp. fresh basil leaves, torn

- 1-2 tbsp. fresh parsley, chopped
- Salt and pepper, to taste

Directions:

1. Place all the meatball ingredients except the oil into a medium bowl.
2. Using your hands, mix well and form into meatballs.
3. Place the oil into a stock pot, place over a medium heat and add the meatballs, browning on all sides.
4. Remove the meatballs from the pan.
5. Add more oil to the pan if needed and then add the onion. Cook for five minutes until soft.
6. Add the remaining soup ingredients, stir well then cook for 10 minutes.
7. Return the meatballs to the pan and simmer for a few minutes to warm through.
8. Serve and enjoy.

Nutrition:

Calories: 331;

Protein: 14.3g;

Carbs: 14.4g;

Fat: 30.3g

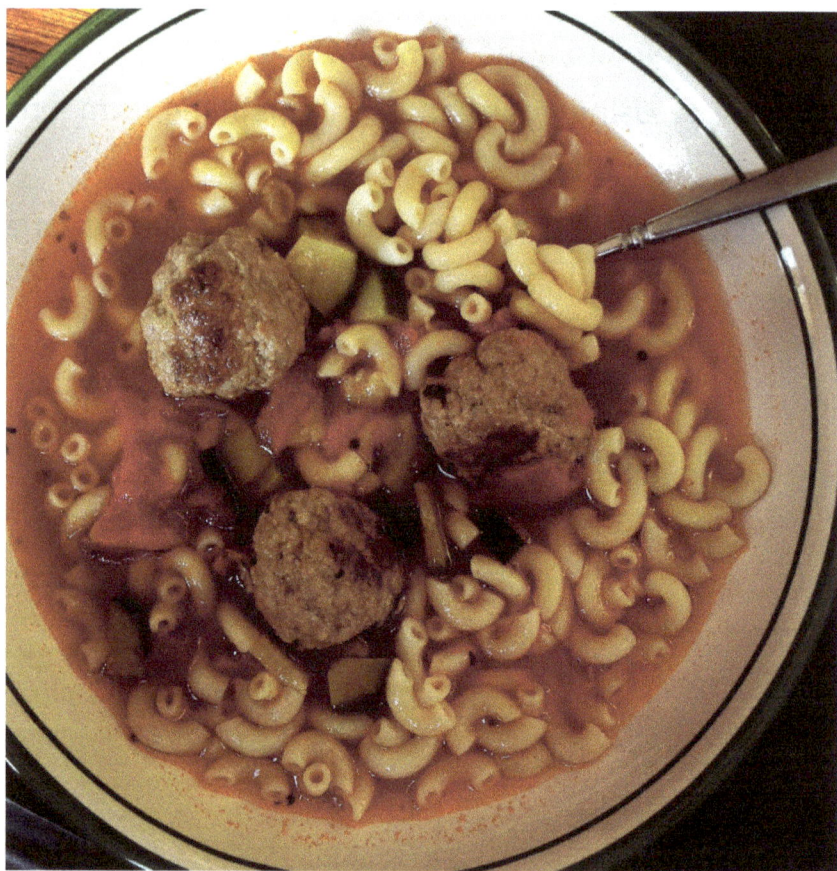

Tuscan White Bean Soup with Sausage and Kale

Preparation Time: 10 minutes

Cooking Time: 40 minutes

Servings: 6

Ingredients:

- ¼ cup extra virgin olive oil
- 1 lb. hot sausage,
- 1 onion, chopped
- 1 carrot, chopped
- 1 stalk celery, chopped
- 2 cloves garlic, chopped
- ½ lb. kale, stems removed and chopped
- 4 cups chicken broth
- 1 x 28 oz. can cannelloni beans, rinsed and drained
- 1 tsp. rosemary, dried
- 1 bay leaf
- ¼ tsp. pepper
- Salt, to taste
- ½ cup shredded parmesan

Directions:

1. Find a stock pot, pop over a medium heat and add the oil.
2. Cook the sausage until browned on all sides.

3. Throw in the onion, carrot, celery and garlic then cook for a further five minutes.

4. Add the kale and stir through.

5. Next add the broth, beans, rosemary and bay leaf.

6. Stir well, bring to the boil then cover with the lid.

7. Turn down the heat then simmer for 30 minutes.

8. Serve and enjoy.

Nutrition:

Calories: 551;

Protein: 36.3g;

Carbs: 33.4g;

Fat: 30.3g

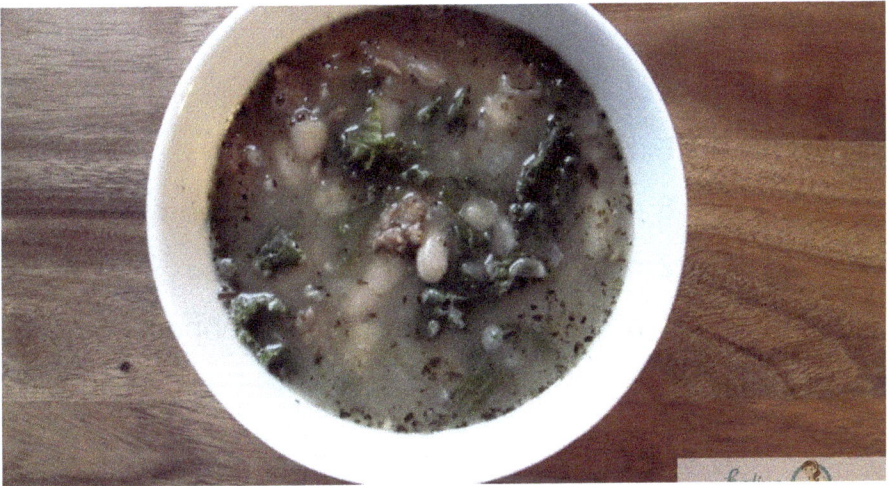

Vegetable Soup

Preparation Time: 10 minutes

Cooking Time: 45 minutes

Servings: 4

Ingredients:

- Extra virgin olive oil, to taste
- 8 oz. sliced baby Bella mushrooms
- 2 medium-size zucchinis, sliced
- 1 bunch flat leaf parsley, chopped
- 1 red onion, chopped
- 2 garlic cloves, chopped
- 2 celery ribs, chopped
- 2 carrots, peeled, chopped
- 2 golden potatoes, peeled, diced
- 1 tsp. ground coriander
- 1/2 tsp. turmeric powder
- 1/2 tsp. sweet paprika
- 1/2 tsp. thyme
- Salt and pepper

- 1 x 32 oz. can whole peeled tomatoes
- 2 bay leaves
- 6 cups turkey or vegetable broth
- 1 x 15 oz. can garbanzo beans, rinsed and drained
- Juice and zest of 1 lime
- 1/3 cup toasted pine nuts, optional

Directions:

1. Grab a large stockpot, add a tbsp. of olive oil and pop over a medium heat.
2. Add the mushrooms and cook for five minutes, stirring often.
3. Remove from the pan and pop to one side.
4. Add the sliced zucchini and cook for another five minutes. Remove from the pan.
5. Add more oil and add the parsley, onions, garlic, celery, carrots and potatoes. Stir through the spices, salt and pepper.
6. Cook for five minutes until the veggies are softening.
7. Add the tomatoes, bay leaves and broth then bring to a boil.

8. Cover and cook on medium low for 15 minutes.

9. Remove the lid and add the garbanzo beans, mushrooms and zucchini.

10. Heat then serve and enjoy.

Nutrition:

Calories: 123;

Protein: 12.3g;

Carbs: 33.4g;

Fat: 19.3g

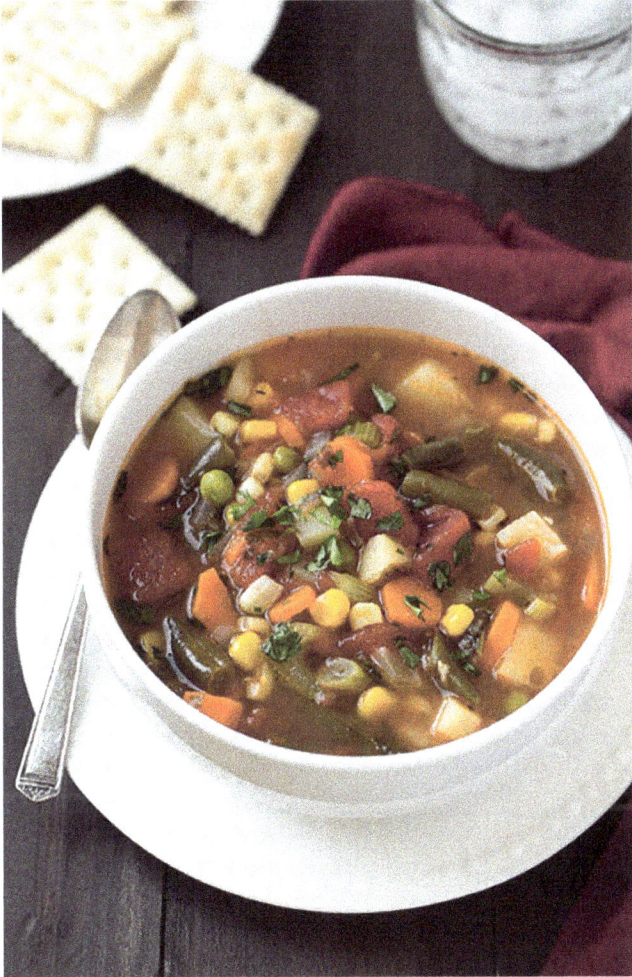

Sweet Yogurt Bulgur Bowl

Preparation Time: 10 minutes

Cooking Time: 0 minutes

Servings: 4

Ingredients:

- 1 cup grapes, halved
- ½ cup bulgur, cooked
- ¼ cup celery stalk, chopped
- 2 oz walnuts, chopped
- ¼ cup plain yogurt
- ½ tsp. ground cinnamon

Directions:

1. Mix grapes with bulgur, celery stalk, and walnut
2. Then add plain yogurt and ground cinnamon.
3. Stir the mixture with the help of the spoon and transfer in the serving bowls.

Nutrition:

Calories: 123;

Protein: 12.3g;

Carbs: 33.4g;

Fat: 19.3g

Spring Farro Plate

Preparation Time: 15 minutes

Cooking Time: 0 minutes

Servings: 6

Ingredients:

- 1 cup farro, cooked
- 2 cups baby spinach
- 2 grapefruits, roughly chopped
- 2 tbsp. balsamic vinegar
- ¼ tsp. white pepper
- 1 tbsp. olive oil

Directions:

1. Mix baby spinach and farro in the big bowl.
2. Then add grapefruit and shake the ingredients well.
3. Transfer the mixture in the serving plates and sprinkle with white pepper, olive oil, and balsamic vinegar.

Nutrition:

Calories: 113;

Protein: 12.3g;

Carbs: 33.4g;

Fat: 19.3g

Sorghum Taboule

Preparation Time: 10 minutes

Cooking Time: 0 minutes

Servings: 2

Ingredients:

- 2 oz sorghum, cooked
- 3 oz pumpkin, diced, boiled
- ½ white onion, diced
- 1 date, pitted, chopped
- 1 tbsp. avocado oil
- ½ tsp. liquid honey
- 2 oz Feta, crumbled

Directions:

1. Put sorghum, pumpkin, onion, and date in the big bowl.
2. Then sprinkle the ingredients with avocado oil and liquid honey. Stir well.
3. Transfer the cooked taboule in the serving plates and top with crumbled feta.

Nutrition:

Calories: 123;

Protein: 12.3g;

Carbs: 33.4g;

Fat: 19.3g

Roasted Sorghum

Preparation Time: 10 minutes

Cooking Time: 15 minutes

Servings: 4

Ingredients:

- 1 tbsp. avocado oil
- ½ cup sorghum, cooked
- 1 carrot, diced
- 2 tbsp. dried parsley
- ½ tsp. dried oregano
- 2 tbsp. cream cheese

Directions:

1. Heat avocado oil and add the carrot.
2. Roast it for 5 minutes.
3. Then add cooked sorghum, parsley, oregano, and cream cheese.
4. Roast the meal for 10 minutes on low heat. Stir it from time to time to avoid burning.

Nutrition:

Calories: 123;

Protein: 2.3g;

Carbs: 3.4g;

Fat: 9.3g

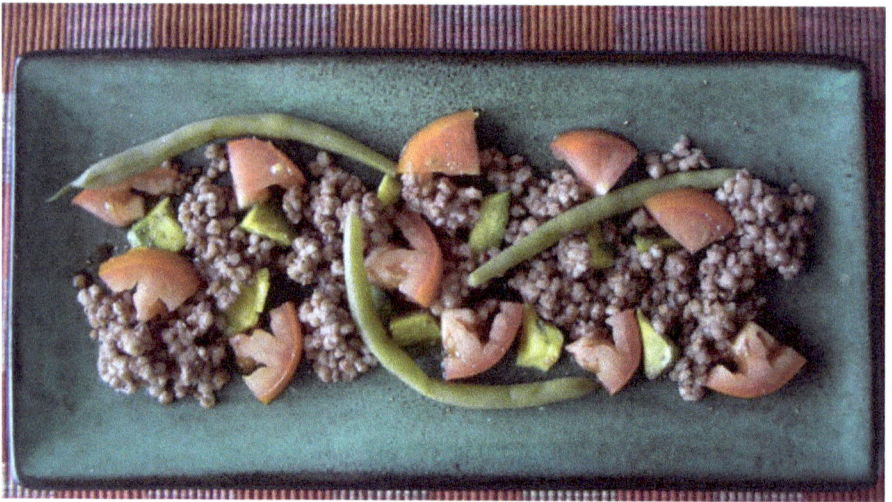

Sorghum Stew

Preparation Time: 10 minutes

Cooking Time: 25 minutes

Servings: 5

Ingredients:

- 1 cup sorghum
- ½ cup ground sausages
- ½ cup tomatoes
- 1 jalapeno pepper, chopped
- ½ cup bell pepper, chopped
- 4 cups chicken stock

Directions:

1. Roast the sausages for 5 minutes in the saucepan.
2. Then add tomatoes, jalapeno, and bell pepper.
3. Cook the ingredients for 10 minutes.
4. After this, add sorghum and chicken stock and boil the stew for 10 minutes more.

Nutrition:

Calories: 127;

Protein: 12.3g;

Carbs: 13.4g;

Fat: 19.3g

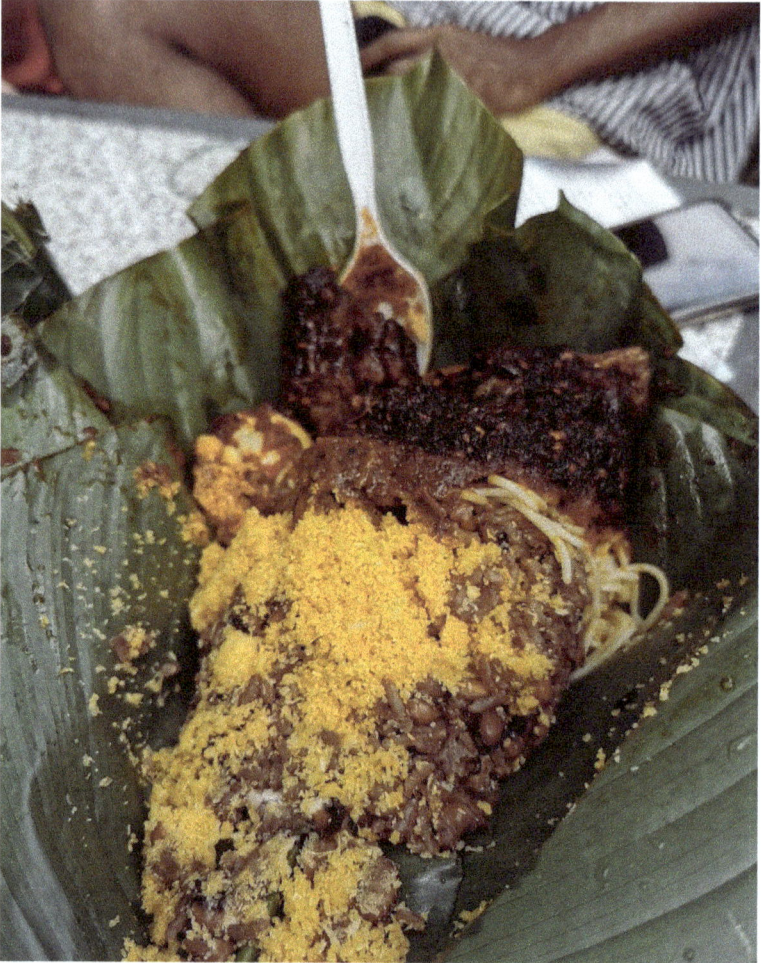

Sorghum Salad

Preparation Time: 10 minutes

Cooking Time: 10 minutes

Servings: 3

Ingredients:

- 3 oz butternut squash, chopped
- ¼ cup sorghum
- ¼ cup fresh cilantro, chopped
- 1 tsp. ground cumin
      cups water
- 2 tbsp. organic canola oil
- 2 tbsp. apple cider vinegar

Directions:

1. Put sorghum and butternut squash in the saucepan.
2. Add water and cook for 10 minutes.
3. Then cool the ingredients and transfer in the salad bowl.
4. Add cilantro, ground cumin, organic canola oil, and apple cider vinegar.
5. Stir the meal well.

Nutrition:

Calories: 123;

Protein: 12.3g;

Carbs: 16.4g;

Fat: 19.3g

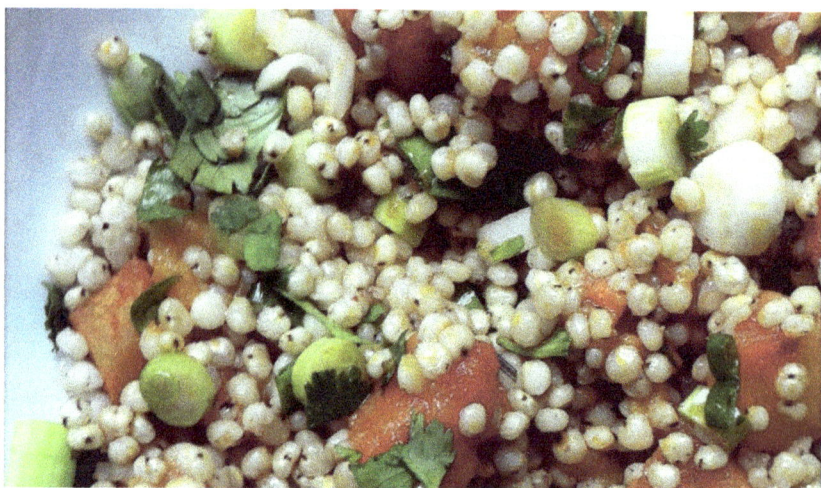

www.ingramcontent.com/pod-product-compliance
Lightning Source LLC
Chambersburg PA
CBHW050755030426
42336CB00012B/1826